Developing Assertiveness Skills for Health and Social Care Professionals

Author

Writer on Health and Social Care Management

Specialist Paediatric Speech and Language Therapist,
Somerset Partnership

Foreword by

Pam Enderby MBE, PhD, FRCSLT
Professor of Community Rehabilitation,
University of Sheffield

Radcliffe Publishing
London • New York

Radcliffe Publishing Ltd
33–41 Dallington Street
London
EC1V 0BB
United Kingdom

www.radcliffehealth.com

British Library Cataloguing in Publication Data

A catalogue record for this book is available from the British Library.

ISBN-13: 978 184619 977 6

The paper used for the text pages of this book is FSC® certified. FSC (The Forest Stewardship Council®) is an international network to promote responsible management of the world's forests.

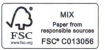

Typeset by Phoenix Photosetting, Chatham, Kent
Printed and bound by TJ International Ltd, Padstow, Cornwall

Contents

Foreword

The many and significant changes to international health, education and social care systems over the past few years are likely to continue as countries are faced with the challenges of financial restrictions at the same time as the need for expanding health and social care structures. This in response to increasing numbers of children with significant disabilities surviving longer, the needs of the more elderly population, greater expectations and rapidly changing technology. All of these will have a substantial impact on the technical and personal skills required by allied health professionals.

One thing is certain. All those involved in health, education and social care will see substantial changes during their time employed within their profession. They will need continually to consider and amend their contribution, develop their skills and respond to new knowledge and technology in order to collaborate effectively in different settings and to meet the changing needs. This will require professional confidence and competence of a different style and nature from what has been required before. More individuals will be working independently, without the security of a prescribed management structure; many will be working with and responsible for assistants and volunteers. They will need to ensure that they comply with the professional standards set by the regulatory authorities and legislative structure. This demands a greater emphasis on clarity of communication, explicit awareness of competence and the confidence to assert one's knowledge, as well as a surety of one's limitations.

This book will help professionals to develop their assertiveness skills in order to equip them for the changing world and manage the many demands and stresses in a positive and productive manner. The objective of the book is that readers will increase their competence and confidence, which will be of benefit to themselves, their colleagues and, most importantly, their clients.

Pam Enderby MBE, PhD, FRCSLT
Professor of Community Rehabilitation, University of Sheffield
June 2013

About the author

Annie Phillips has written professionally about health and health management since she qualified as a speech and language therapist in 1978. She has over 30 years' NHS experience in primary and secondary care as a clinician and a manager.

Her first 10 years as a speech and language therapist, specialising in adult neurology and elderly care, led to the research and publication of an international dysphasia/dementia screening test, presented at the 1986 British Aphasiology Conference. She has won various prizes and awards for her subsequent work, and in the 1990s was a finalist in the Medeconomics Good Management Awards and regional winner in a national British Institute of Management competition on Change Management.

She worked as a practice and fund manager for a five-partner training GP practice in central Brighton from 1989 to 1998; from then as an independent health advisor, trainer and management consultant to general practice and PCTs. As a management consultant, her interest focused on organisational analysis and the development of healthy organisations, with an emphasis on finding ways to manage stresses and conflicts, understanding and alleviating dysfunctional communication and developing effective management strategies.

In 2000, she returned to clinical work as a paediatric speech and language therapist, and continues in this work to date.

Throughout her career she has written extensively for the therapy, medical and management press on contemporary management issues for a range of publications, including the *Health Service Journal, Community Care, Pulse, Medi-Economics, Doctor, Primary Care Manager* and Croner Publications, with a focus on healthcare politics and clinical management. Her first book, *The Business Planning Toolkit: a workbook for the primary care team*, was published in 2002 (Radcliffe Publishing), and was swiftly followed by three others, including the *Assertiveness* book that is now being updated.

Annie can be contacted via the publishers.

Acknowledgements

Thanks to all those family and friends who have supported me in my own personal development: all my favourite people (you know who you are!). Your love, friendship, support and ideas have sustained me over the years.

I also wish to record my thanks and debt of gratitude to Dr Pam Enderby – whom I met first in the early 1980s, whose work inspired me to begin thinking about the importance of evidence-based working; and subsequently the partners at St Peter's Medical Centre, Brighton – especially Dr Howard Carter – for the help, encouragement and valuable advice gained during my employment through the 1990s. On to all my PCT, training and management colleagues – some of whom were inspirational; all of whom challenged my thinking. Without all of these people, my journey into understanding the theory of clinical management would not have been possible. It is in these jobs I really learned that management was a professional field in its own right, with academic rigour, and not simply an add-on to clinical work.

And on to this decade, to those colleagues too numerous to mention whose wise counsel challenges me to continue learning – including all those who continue to teach me as I work with them; the current bunch being the Somerset Integrated Therapy Team, especially – but not exclusively – my dear friends Tash, Lyndsey and Lauren, and for the management team who tirelessly support me in my process! Special thanks to Fanny Rowe, whose devolved management style and expert leadership allow us therapists to feel safe, while encouraging and supporting our creativity and developing clinical skills.

I want to thank all those whose thoughts and ideas have, over the years, found their way into my subconscious, so they are now indistinguishable from my own. In this vein, if I have unintentionally misquoted anyone, my apologies. I have attempted to give sources of work where possible, but apologise if, inadvertently, I have failed to record it correctly. Should you note any queries, errors or omissions, please contact the publisher. Special thanks too to my editors, Jamie Etherington and Elisabeth Doyle, for all their hard work and for dealing so sensitively with any changes required; and finally to the typesetters, Phoenix Photosetting, for making the book look fabulous.

Finally, my very special thanks as always to my partner Lin, for her love, encouragement and support; for her thoughtful additions, insightful editing; and for gracefully giving me the time out from our family commitments to continue writing.

Introduction

What is assertiveness, and can anyone learn to be assertive? Why do those in the caring professions in particular need to be assertive? Why is the focus on women learning the skills, not men? What about aggression? How can I train my clients to be more assertive? These questions have often been asked of me. People are anxious about assertiveness – they mistakenly equate it with selfishness, aggression or a lack of humour. Others feel they are not brave, or brash, enough to learn and implement the skills, let alone teach them to others. But it is possible to learn to be assertive. With time, patience and practice anyone can learn how to be assertive.

To be assertive is to communicate clearly, honestly and directly, without avoidance or resorting to manipulative or aggressive behaviour. The aim of this book is to explain what assertiveness is and how to be assertive, and to explore the advantages of using assertiveness as the main tool of effective, advanced communication skills in health and social care settings. We take a look at assertiveness as an interpersonal communication skill, which is required to communicate more effectively. My reader is anyone who works in health or social care as a manager or clinician, anyone who deals with people – staff, the public, clients or patients – on a daily basis, and needs these dealings to be thoughtful, effective and stress free. The target market is all those who work in care settings: acute medicine, primary care and the community; any member of the care team, with or without a management role, who wants to understand how to develop their relationships with their colleagues, clients, patients and managers – anyone who needs to:
➤ understand and alleviate barriers to effective communication
➤ manage the stresses and conflicts that arise between people
➤ develop effective clinical and people skills.

I write with an assumption that we are working towards an integrated model of working across all sectors, hence my inclusion of all care settings across the public and private sector. I have endeavoured to use inclusive language, so have used both 'patient' and 'client' to describe recipients of our services, with recognition that the term 'patient' can be problematic. The dictionary definition ('able to accept or tolerate delays, problems, or suffering without becoming annoyed or anxious'; 'a person receiving or registered to receive medical treatment') places people very much in an inferior position: in receipt of, rather than determining, their care. 'Client', referring to 'a person or organisation using the services of a professional person', is, I feel, preferable.

Many care systems are still set up with a medical model bias. Although the majority of healthcare training institutes (medicine/nursing/allied health professionals) include material relating to the social model of disability, and the integration of social with medical interventions is more appreciated than it used to be, in the UK we are sadly still trailing behind in a patient-centred delivery – which integrates working advocates. The UK performance in patient-centred care rated seventh in a comparison with six other European countries, despite achieving the second highest status overall when including all other parameters (clinical effectiveness, speed of delivery, etc.).[1] This needs to change.

However, 'patient' as a term is included in recognition that many readers work with people whose physical ill-health is the main reason for them presenting. The terminology portrays a medical power-base that I am not always entirely comfortable with: it takes patients away from being central in their own recovery process. The social (bio-psycho-social) model of healthcare more frequently in use now recognises that in many circumstances – in pre-natal and dementia care, psychological therapy and social care, for example – the people using these services are not physically 'ill' but in need of support through a process of change.

The publication of this book is timely. The recently published draft report from the Commission on Improving Dignity in Care for Older People (2012) has prompted reflections and discussions on professionalism across the health and social care workforce. We are debating what goes wrong, how to right it, the need to behave in a professional way, what professionalism looks like. The Health Professions Council has identified 'treating patients and service users with respect, communicating clearly, involving people in decisions about their own care, keeping accurate records of treatments and interventions' as fundamental to good professional practice.[2] These have been reported on recently, and I want this book to contribute to the debate and help sharpen up ideas of professionalism in healthcare.

This book has a second, companion volume: *Developing Leadership Skills for Health and Social Care Professionals*. The two should be read in tandem,

---

1   Ham C, Dixon A, Brooks B. *Transforming the Delivery of Health and Social Care: the case for fundamental change*. King's Fund; 2012.

2   Health Professions Council. *Fitness to Practise Annual Report 2008* and *Standards of Conduct, Performance and Ethics 2008*. Also: Health Professions Council. *Professionalism in Nursing, Midwifery and the Allied Health Professions in Scotland: a report to the coordinating council for the NMAHP Contribution to the Healthcare Quality Strategy for NHS Scotland*. Health Professions Council; 2012.

as in this second volume I include information about the broader aspects of communication – understanding ourselves and others, our motivations, interests and perspectives – to encourage the development of interpersonal skills and keep our observational and caring skills sharp.

All of us working in health should keep in mind a motivation of caring and helping, be able to recognise, support and empathise with distress, foster feelings of warmth and kindness, develop qualities of patience and tolerance, and be able to look at difficulties in order to learn from them and develop wisdom. We need, in healthcare, to work with intellectual rigour, emotional intelligence and compassion, and should apply these qualities when dealing with others, be it patients or staff. In this volume we find the usual sections on learning the skills of assertiveness, as well as the personal and professional skills needed to navigate successfully through a clinical career. This book challenges the reader to reconstruct their communication and behave more confidently and equally. It provokes and encourages the reader to invest in his or her own personal and professional development. I analyse some of the barriers to good communication in healthcare, and the skills we need to develop professionally: confidence, self-awareness and development of critical faculties.

The book is divided into four sections. The first and second sections describe basic assertiveness skills and how to apply them in difficult situations, including information on giving constructive, kindly and clear feedback to patients and their relatives (in challenging circumstances) and managing conflict and disputes. We unpick some of the skills in more detail: how to negotiate; how to deal with making and refusing requests; how to manage conflict and aggression.

In the third section we explore some of the clinical challenges, including broadening our understanding of patient rights and the relevance of this in the new healthcare climate of patient empowerment. We discuss setting boundaries in treatment, and what we can offer in the present climate; informing patients of their choices, and also what we can and cannot be expected to deliver. We examine some of the models for working with this, how to break difficult news with understanding, expertise and compassion, and support patients with learning the skills to manage their own recovery process. It is salutary to learn that amongst speech and language therapists, 56% do not feel comfortable or confident discussing end of life issues with patients.[3] They will not be alone, and this section aims to address some of these concerns.

In the last section we apply some of our learned skills: we look at using assertiveness in planning and managing our work through goal setting and change management.

---

3   Royal College of Speech & Language Therapists. *Bulletin*. December 2012. Available at: www.rcslt.org

At the end of each chapter I have included some summary points to assist the reader in reflecting on the concepts explored and identifying any learning needs.

Assertive people achieve success as they bring themselves into the best focus possible. They take control of situations. They take responsibility to use all their capabilities. They do not avoid conflict or difficulties or ignore problems. They take charge and confront inefficiency, unfairness, mediocrity or poor conduct with honesty and clarity, without which they could not achieve in life or work. Assertive people face their insecurities, and learn how to cope with authority. They allow themselves to make mistakes, knowing that assurance comes with experience. They know there is no such thing as perfection in people, remembering that good intentions are as important as any other quality. They listen, ask questions, take advice and then act. Successful people do not leave anything to chance; they take charge of their life. And that is what being assertive is all about.

Annie Phillips
June 2013

Section 1

Assertiveness skills

Aggressive

➤ Is angry, defensive, and competitive.
➤ Puts others down.
➤ Has low self-esteem.
➤ Finds themselves in the middle of conflict, confrontation, attacks.
➤ Overreacts.
➤ Their communication can lead to others feeling hurt, humiliated and resentful.
➤ Releases anger at the expense of others.

Manipulative

➤ Gets their own way through flirting, pandering to egos.
➤ Has low self-esteem.
➤ Is indirect, subtle.
➤ Fears exposure (it is safer to control and manipulate than to risk rejection).
➤ Is devious, appearing to think highly of others but with an undercurrent of disapproval.
➤ May deny if others attempt to clarify.

Assertive

➤ Says what they want without resorting to anger or manipulation.
➤ Respects people.
➤ Accepts their own positive and negative feelings.
➤ Is more tolerant, less judgemental.
➤ Takes responsibility for themselves, their feelings and reactions.
➤ Acknowledges their own needs.
➤ Asks directly and honestly.
➤ Risks refusal.
➤ Has good self-esteem.
➤ Is not dependent on others.
➤ Sets their own limits and boundaries.

We are all a mix of behavioural styles, and our history and genes dictate our personality traits to some extent, but this book aims to show how you can communicate more honestly, openly and directly, and avoid the manipulation, anger and passivity that may be a more habitual stance. Some of the early work on assertiveness is to try to gauge the ways you habitually respond in a difficult, domestic situation.

How would you respond?

A friend asks you a favour:

'Since you're going to be away for the week, I'm wondering if I could borrow your car? Our second car is out of action and my wife needs one to take the kids to school.'

You do not really want to lend your car. How do you reply?

Passive: 'Sure, ok.' [*subtext:* 'Of course I don't want to lend my car, I don't want the wear and tear, worry about X's driving, and am not even sure if I have got the time to sort the insurance. However, it is more important to me to be liked/kind.']

Aggressive: 'You're kidding! No way, I haven't got time to sort this out.'

Assertive: 'I'm sorry you have a problem this week. However, I don't lend my car out. How about trying X, they're a really reliable and cheap car hire firm just down the road from you. I can run you there if you like.' [*subtext:* 'I like you and wish I could help out. However, this is your problem, not mine. But I am not such a poor friend that I can't go some way to help you.']

All of us have the right to be treated with respect, to be listened to and taken seriously. We have the right to set our own priorities and choose for ourselves. We have the right to express our own feelings and opinions – including saying 'no' – without fear. We have the right to make mistakes.

Moving on from the domestic, it is especially important for us care workers to use assertiveness skills because we do care: we care inherently for, the patients/clients, staff, the organisations we work for. We can therefore feel very guilty when we do not, or are unable to, live up to the caring image. We often think of ourselves as indispensable: our work can involve sacrifice; we often find it hard to delegate. We do not want to offend: it is extremely easy for us to feel guilty. Consider the following scenarios.

➤ You feel guilty about keeping to time boundaries – you need to be available to your patients/clients and colleagues at all times.

➤ You do not move to a more stimulating or rewarding job because you know there will be difficulties recruiting your replacement.

➤ You do not push your staff as hard as you should because you can empathise with their difficulties around increasing service demands.

➤ You reluctantly accept a new system of working that you have reservations about because you do not want to offend the colleagues/your manager who is enthusiastic about it.

People who consistently behave in this way will overstretch and exhaust themselves. They are taking care of everyone else but themselves, at huge cost to their own physical and mental well-being. They think themselves indispensible, and soon 'burn out'.

Here is a useful exercise to do with a friend or sympathetic colleague.

EXERCISE 1

The compassion trap

Using the columns below, list those things that you do for other people because they ask you, not because you want to do them or accept they are part of your role.

Work	Friendships	Home

For example:

Work	Friendships	Home
Always make the coffee Work overtime almost every day Take the on call every Christmas	Always lend my car Talk with X for hours on end even through I have other family demands	Do lion's share of the housework Go to parent's evening every time

➤ Swap lists.
➤ Role-play the situation. Your part is to say 'no' politely but firmly.
➤ What does the 'no' feel like?

If you feel you need more practice, *see* Chapter 7, Making and refusing requests.

How to change

To be assertive is not to behave selfishly – it is about responsible self-care. Assertive people recognise their own limits, manage their own resources so as to work effectively, without resentment, and are able to call a halt before they burn out. They give themselves time to rest and replenish their energies, so that when they do give once more they do so with sustainable strength and enthusiasm.

Do you:
➤ find delegation difficult
➤ assume responsibility for other people's needs
➤ deny people equal rights of interaction
➤ organise other people's lives

➤ make decisions for friends, family and co-workers
➤ assume people cannot manage by themselves?

Here, you are taking inappropriate responsibility for others' lives. Women in particular are reluctant to relinquish work-based power, as it can be one of the only areas of their life where they hold it. If this is the case, by taking more power for yourself assertively you will feel able to give up this strong manipulative hold and claim real equality.

You will still be able to show compassion, love and care to others, but the choice will be yours: you are not compelled always to put others' needs before your own to maintain your own self-worth.

YOUR RIGHTS

We all have needs, rights, opinions and choices. Because of cultural pressures, those in less powerful positions can find it difficult to acknowledge that they are entitled to these, but the paradox is that they understand, acknowledge and fulfil other people's all the time! When we acknowledge that we too have certain rights, we set ourselves free from the dependence on others for their approval.

➤ We fear disapproval because it threatens our sense of self.
➤ We may have felt hurt and unloved when younger.
➤ This fear (of losing love) can then easily shift to other respected, or authority figures in our lives – especially those at work.
➤ We want to be liked, and in anticipating disapproval we avoid stating our needs.

Consider the following.

Hazel is a successful and respected emergency care manager, working in A&E. She pioneered a departmental move, and the development of some new, innovative patient services. She has acted as the catalyst for a lot of positive change. She has decided, after much consideration, that she wishes to resign and move on, after only 18 months in the post.

Her employers plead with her. They ask her why she is leaving; they are concerned that the department will collapse without her. Hazel feels caught in a trap. She feels the need of the staff and her employers and is concerned that she will appear selfish if she leaves so soon. Perhaps she should carry on for another few years. She feels guilt and sympathy for her colleagues left to manage 'by themselves'. Eventually she states her position assertively. She acknowledges the department's position, and explains that she has enjoyed bringing in the innovations she has and has contributed and learned a lot. However, she wants to develop other skills now, that she feels are better suited to another role. The others hear her and respect her clarity and decision; Hazel leaves feeling satisfied that she has made the right choice.

Hazel was allowing herself to have needs. She needed time, a change of scene and a different challenge. Had she stayed in post, she would have become stale, possibly resentful. The explanation she gave to her colleagues demonstrated her concern for her workplace, but also showed that she too had needs and other plans that she wished to fulfil. She chose for herself assertively.

Anne Dickson[6] sets out what has come to be known as a Bill of Rights – pin it up somewhere.

I have the right to:

Be treated with respect

Set my own priorities

Ask for what I want

Be listened to and taken seriously

Set my own goals

Say 'no' without feeling guilty

Express my own feelings and opinions

Make mistakes

Ask for, and obtain information from professionals

To receive criticism in my own way

Get what I pay for

Choose for myself

---

6   Dickson, Charlesworth, note 5 above.

Examine these rights in more detail. What do they mean for us health and social care workers, within or outside the organisations we work for?

1   I have the right to be treated with respect

In a system where both doctors and medical managers regard power inequalities as natural, necessary and beneficial, this is hard. Doctors tend to attach little value to having a supportive superior, and back a medical ascendancy model of management. The present culture may work for medics, but it certainly does not work for the co-workers.

Within this system it is very difficult for a non-medic to have and offer opinions. It is easy to forget that what we feel and what we have to say as an intelligent and informed individual counts, as there is always someone ready and willing to put you in your place. We need to remember in these circumstances that our own needs and opinions matter too. Being treated with respect means:

➤ being noticed: there are many occasions when the opinions of the less medically qualified are not sought; they are ignored
➤ others may not agree with what you have to say, but you have a right to a voice and may be able to offer a valuable additional perspective
➤ that your time is valued and appreciated, for example, people cannot always assume that they can talk with you at *their* convenience.

2   I have the right to set my own priorities

If you are feeling disempowered, it is very easy to let others lead your agenda. Set your own priorities. One might be the need to set aside time for yourself: see yourself as someone who deserves as much time, effort and energy as your family, your colleagues, your employers, the patients/clients. If you permit yourself the right to look after your own life, the need for others to speak *for* you is removed. Once you give yourself permission to set you own priorities, the balance of power is redressed if someone pressures you to follow their agenda.

Let us take another example.

Kate is a practice manager who has allocated some time in her day to review the practice accounts. The practice is busy dealing with a flu epidemic, but among other pressures and deadlines, Kate has to review these accounts prior to a meeting with the accountant the following day. She wants to present a summary to the senior partner at their lunchtime review. When she arrives in her office, one of the partners rushes in to greet her in a panic. He asks her if she could possibly cover reception, as they are short – and it is a Monday morning. Kate acknowledges the partner's difficulties, but reasserts her need and wish to continue with the work she is doing. She will, however, do her utmost to obtain locum cover, and picks up the phone instantly to set this in motion.

Kate, as a fellow professional, has set her own limits and priorities for the day, she need not allow the senior partner to organise her, as she is capable of organising herself.

3   I have the right to ask for what I want

Here you establish your right to identify and communicate your needs as an equal. It is easy, especially when you are newly qualified or new to an organisation, to feel that you do not matter, and to be in awe of others who seem much older and more experienced. All of us need to remember that we too have the right to ask for what we want, and to ask for information or clarification if we do not understand.

➤ Allow yourself to communicate your needs to others, remembering of course that you cannot always expect those needs to be met – allow yourself room for negotiation.

➤ Never accept substandard accommodation to work in. Everyone working in the public sector is entitled to accommodation that is quiet, free from distractions and suitably furnished. Refuse to work in unsuitable premises; it is only by doing this that some respect will eventually be shown to you and your profession.

➤ Never allow yourself to accept rude, aggressive or undermining behaviour.

➤ If you do not voice your concerns, your work will be undervalued.

➤ Ask for what you want – you have nothing to lose. If you do not ask, others will not know.

4   I have the right to be listened to and taken seriously

What you say may not, of course, always be right, but you do have a right to air your opinions. Do not allow your age or (apparent) lack of professional standing to belittle you. What you have to say is important to you otherwise you would not be saying it – whether you are acting in a professional capacity or not. You have the right too to make statements that others may deem illogical, without justification.

5   I have the right to set my own goals

➤ Make your own choices when decisions need to be made.

➤ Do not allow others automatically to chose for you.

➤ Set your own goals, your own standards and limits.

➤ Ask for that help if you need it.

It is very easy to fall into the trap of giving others the power to make our decisions for us. When we were children, we looked to our parents to make important decisions on our behalf – our education, and often our choice of career, was a parental choice and not entirely our own. Once you are an adult, give yourself the right and the responsibility of choosing for yourself: you are capable of planning and controlling your own life.

6   I have the right to say 'no' without feeling guilty

If you consistently put others' needs before your own, you fall into the compassion trap mentioned earlier. Allow yourself to balance out your own needs with those of other people. Make your own decisions and choices, which includes saying 'no' periodically to demands made on you. If you are being asked to do something that you feel unable or unwilling to do, think again before automatically agreeing.

7   I have the right to express my own feelings and opinions

➤ You have the right to hold an opinion, have feelings and emotions about issues, and to express them appropriately.
➤ Do not allow others to manipulate you or try to make you change your mind.
➤ Do not allow others to deny you your feelings.
➤ Be ready to stand by your own opinions when others try to belittle you.

The passive person would automatically concede, and agree with another opinion to preserve the peace. An aggressive person would present his or her opinions dogmatically, denying others the right to share theirs. The assertive person respects another's opinions and feelings, while acknowledging that he or she holds a (possibly) differing view.

8   I have the right to make mistakes

Mistakes are acceptable – everyone makes them. The world does not collapse when we make one wrong move. Acknowledge the mistake and start afresh. In this way your self-esteem and confidence in yourself is retained. You also have the right to change your mind: this is part of taking responsibility for your own decisions and dealing with the consequences; it may also show flexibility and that your thinking has advanced.

9   I have the right to ask for and get information from professionals

Remember your individual, or consumer, rights when faced with professionals who often withhold information to retain power or authority. Do not be afraid to admit that you do not understand, as often an acknowledgement of your own weaknesses will be met with sympathy and respect. Admit to ignorance, confusion or not knowing, and feel confident to ask for clarification or for more information. Ask clearly and confidently, avoiding subtleties and suggestions. A clear, direct question should be met with an equally clear, respectful response.

10   I have the right to receive criticism in my own way

Allow yourself the right to accept criticism if you feel that it is fair; but ask for clarification or example if you feel the criticism is unjustified. In this way you need not be totally demolished by personal comments or criticisms. You do not need to take unjustified criticism on board.

11   I have the right to get what I pay for

You have a right not only to return goods that are faulty, but also to reflect that you deserve fair treatment from people whose services you have requested. If you attend a course that you feel was poor value for money, say so! If your employer promises to set aside an hour to discuss a problem then takes phone calls throughout the discussion, air your grievance! If an informal 'contract' has been set up between two people, it is unfair for one not to keep to his or her side of the agreement. You deserve better treatment.

12   I have the right to choose for myself

The assertive person successfully assesses his or her own behaviour and thus releases him- or herself from dependence on the opinions of others.

➤ You have the right to chose whether or not to get involved with someone.
➤ You have the right to chose privacy.
➤ You have the right to be alone and independent.
➤ You have the right to be assertive.

EXERCISE 2

> In the left hand column, list your own needs, the favourite things in your life that you enjoy.

For example, I like watching daytime TV/I like living alone/I like reading in bed. On the right, list any people who impose on those activities and say why you feel you cannot do them.

I like eating lunch alone	There is pressure on me to eat with the team in the staffroom

You can also chose when, where and if you wish to be assertive: do not berate yourself if you cannot, or chose not to, do so.

Some blocks to assertiveness

What prevents people from being assertive? Many people are anxious about acquiring a new skill, or may procrastinate. Others are frightened. They may have a fear of rejection, of hurting others, of violence, of failure, or of financial insecurity (people are less assertive and more compliant in an economic downturn, when they may fear losing their job). There may be few assertive role models around, so there may be a lack of opportunity to see and acquire the skills. For some, they may have cultural, philosophical or religious beliefs that prevent an interest – assertive behaviour can be seen as threatening or selfish in some cultures. If you have emotional blocks such as these, try to question them, and imagine the real consequences of behaving assertively.

Remember that to be assertive is also to behave compassionately – behaving compassionately is not submissive, nor does it mean simply giving in to what other people want, which may leave us feeling resentful or needy for their approval. It is never easy to act wisely or compassionately from a position of fear or weakness. Compassion requires thoughtfulness, curiosity and openness, but at times it also requires courage – and these are qualities that we all at times struggle with. Sometimes we have to be brave to be assertive, to stand up to others and say 'no'.

Further help

If any of these scenarios sound familiar, you need someone to be on your side. Some employing organisations offer training; psychological therapists run training courses; the British Association for Counselling and Psychotherapy (BACP)[7] has the names of local counsellors who can help you to move on. Or try your local further education college. There are a myriad of independent consultancy training services, offering training in assertiveness as well as other courses in communication, presentation, coaching and leadership skills.

KEY POINTS

➤ Behaving assertively helps at both a professional and a personal level.

➤ The assertive person takes charge and acts in ways that invite respect, accepting their own limitations and strengths, leading to clearer communication.

➤ Learning to be assertive is seen as an important component in cognitive-behavioural approaches to tackling anger, anxiety, depression and poor self-esteem.

➤ In assertiveness, it is important that we are motivated to behave with good intent, kindness, tolerance and compassion.

---

7   01788 550899; www.bacp.co.uk (accessed May 2013).

➤ The assertive person recognises their needs are no more and no less than others, but equal.

➤ Assertive skills enable us to see our role at work more clearly and cope more readily with feelings of frustration or inadequacy.

➤ To be assertive does not mean that you will always get what you want, or that all your problems will be solved. Assertiveness is one tool among many.

➤ All of us have the right to be treated with respect, to be listened to and to be taken seriously. We have the right to set our on priorities and choose for ourselves. We have the right to express our own feelings and opinions without fear. We have the right to make mistakes.

➤ Compassion requires thoughtfulness, curiosity and openness, but at times it also requires courage – and these are qualities that we all struggle with from time to time. Sometimes we have to be brave to be assertive.

FURTHER READING

Dickson A. *Difficult Conversations: what to say in tricky situations without ruining the relationship*. New ed. Piatkus; 2006.

Dickson A. *The Mirror Within: a new look at sexuality*. Quartet Books; 1985.

Gutmann J. *The Assertiveness Workbook: a plan for busy women*. Sheldon Press; 1993.

Lindenfield G. *Assert Yourself: simple steps to getting what you want*. Thorsons; 2001.

Lindenfield G. *Self Esteem: simple steps to develop self-worth and heal emotional wounds*. Thorsons; 2000.

Lindenfield G. *Super Confidence: simple steps to build self-assurance*. Thorsons; 2000.

APPENDIX 1

Work skill survey

In the list of skills given below, circle the number which best describes how you are at using the skill.

Circle 1 – if you are *never* good at it

Circle 2 – if you are *seldom* good at it

Circle 3 – if you are *sometimes* good at it

Circle 4 – if you are *often* good at it

Circle 5 – if you are *always* good at it

Skills

1 *Listening*   Paying attention to people, trying to understand them and letting them know that you are trying.   1 2 3 4 5

2 *Expressing appreciation*   Letting another person know that you are grateful for something which he or she has done for you.   1 2 3 4 5

3 *Expressing encouragement* Telling someone that he or she should try to do something which they are not sure they can do. 1 2 3 4 5

4 *Asking for help* Asking for someone who is qualified to help you in handling a difficult situation which you have not been able to manage yourself. 1 2 3 4 5

5 *Giving instructions* Clearly explaining to someone how you would like a specific task done. 1 2 3 4 5

6 *Expressing a complaint* Telling someone that he or she is responsible for creating a particular problem for you and attempting to find a particular solution for the problem. 1 2 3 4 5

7 *Responding to others' feelings* Trying to understand what another person is feeling and communicating your understanding to them. 1 2 3 4 5

8 *Responding to persuasion* Carefully considering another person's ideas, weighing them against your own and then deciding which course of action will be best for you in the long run. 1 2 3 4 5

9 *Responding to failure* Figuring out what went wrong and what you can do about it so that you can be more successful in the future. 1 2 3 4 5

10 *Responding to contradictory messages* Recognising and dealing with the confusion that results when a person tells you one thing but says or does things which indicate that he or she means something else. 1 2 3 4 5

11 *Responding to a complaint* Dealing fairly with another person's dissatisfaction with a situation attributed to you. 1 2 3 4 5

12 *Responding to anger* Trying to understand another person's anger and letting him or her know that you are trying. 1 2 3 4 5

13 *Setting a goal* Deciding on what you want to accomplish and judging whether your plan is realistic. 1 2 3 4 5

14 *Gathering information* Deciding what specific information you need and asking the appropriate people for that information. 1 2 3 4 5

15 *Concentrating on a task* Making those preparations that will enable you to get a job done efficiently. 1 2 3 4 5

16 *Evaluating your abilities*   Examining your   1 2 3 4 5
accomplishments fairly and honestly in order to decide
how competent your are in a particular skill.

17 *Preparing for a stressful conversation*   Planning ahead of   1 2 3 4 5
time to present your point of view in a conversation
which may be difficult.

18 *Setting problem priorities*   Deciding which of several   1 2 3 4 5
problems is most urgent and should be worked on first.

19 *Decision making*   Deciding on a realistic course of   1 2 3 4 5
action which you believe will be in your best interest.

20 *Determining responsibility*   Finding out whether your   1 2 3 4 5
actions or the actions of others have caused an event to
occur.

21 *Making requests*   Asking the appropriate person for   1 2 3 4 5
what you need or want.

22 *Relaxation*   Learning to calm down and relax when you   1 2 3 4 5
are tense.

23 *Negotiation*   Arriving at an agreement which is   1 2 3 4 5
satisfactory to you and to another person who has
taken a different position.

24 *Assertiveness*   Standing up for yourself by letting other   1 2 3 4 5
people know what you want, how you feel or what you
think about something.

CHAPTER 2

Women and assertiveness

Women in particular need to develop assertiveness skills. In this and the following chapters it will become apparent why men, for various physiological, psychological, socio-cultural and contextual reasons, find it easier to assert themselves in the workplace.

For the purpose of this book, we need to have some understanding of why women find it harder than men to be assertive, and why so many more woman are being taught assertiveness skills as part of their personal, and emotional, development. Although women more than men can face difficulties when they behave assertively (as it can be perceived as unexpected/unusual behaviour), there are ways we can work with the behaviour to achieve advantage and acceptability.

The fact remains that, over the years, there has been little change in gender stereotyping both in and out of work. Masculine characteristics are deemed to be assertiveness, independence, power and self-reliance, and feminine characteristics are traditionally caring, helpfulness and sharing. The stereotypes are common in many cultures and there can be a backlash if you act out of role. Success at work is usually associated with the male traits of aggression, emotional stability and rationality. If women manifest these behaviours, the fear is they will be seen as tough, hard, unlikable. There is a penalty for women behaving counter to stereotypical expectations, at a cost to success. However, although women more than men can face difficulties when they behave assertively (as it can be perceived as unexpected/unusual behaviour), there are ways we can work with the behaviour to achieve advantage and acceptability.

Although patriarchy puts men in the stronger position, we also need to acknowledge that they are facing a confusing and transforming time, under pressure to reconstruct their masculinity in the face of an increasingly feminised society. Many traditional 'female' qualities and skills are lauded in education and the workplace, facilitation and communication skills in particular. Alpha males are not so lauded: their hyper-competitive, domineering personalities leave them at a disadvantage in modern society, and beta males are taking over.

It is hard, when looking at traditional male behaviour, not to caricature masculinity; particularly when addressing at the more negative traits such as ego, virility, controlling behaviour, misogyny, aggression and violence. This image of masculinity is portrayed in the media and in contemporary culture and, like all stereotypes, in part it is true. There is no doubt these traits feature more in men than in women, as there is no doubt that hormonal, societal and physiological differences exist between the two. While acknowledging this, it is also important to look beyond gender bias to support both men and women with changing their behaviour, and try to look at any differences dispassionately and non-judgmentally.

We know that many men carry an exaggerated sense of pride, and have a terror of being seen as vulnerable.[1] If our aim is to explore, describe and understand rather than demonise some of these less acceptable male behaviours,[2] we need to listen to men more closely. We can then allow them the space to voice their feelings of frustration and vulnerability, and relieve the pressures of duty, expectation and obligation. They will then be in a better place to move on and adapt some more useful skills of relating, and thus affect the well-being of community in the long term.

In terms of assertiveness, we cannot avoid looking at patriarchy and feminism to explain the sense of inferiority that women have; both personal, political and cultural approaches are needed to understand why we behave as we do. And men too, of course, need to learn to adapt their behaviour – particularly non-functional, aggressive behaviour – and work as hard at this as women do to develop a stronger sense of self, and strive to put their needs out there as well.

Research into gender differences is still throwing up questions about whether such differences do occur, or matter, but it is clear that different people do apply different thinking to moral processes, and there is still a clear bias for women and men to have obviously different preferred styles.

Men find being assertive easier as they are, by nature, risk-takers, opportunists; too much ego masquerades as pride and arrogance. Men have been socialised to be proud of themselves and their behaviour, and they find being assertive easier: they are the stronger sex physiologically; they take up more space. Women need to learn to develop their egos: to be prouder of themselves and their success. They cannot change themselves physically, but they can learn symbolically to 'take more space' for themselves, by altering their body language and verbal skills to support a stronger sense of self. Women have a different set of needs.

Carol Gilligan,[3] a psychologist and feminist, has drawn attention to women's need to be more focused on nurturing; men need to be more on problems of competition and the need for regulation through systems of fairness and rights. Women therefore tend to be highly sensitised to the needs of others; our default setting is non-confrontational; we avoid situations where we have

---

1 Bazzano M. Reconstructing masculinity. *Therapy Today*. 2012 Feb. pp. 24–7.
2 Ansbacher HL, Ansbacher R. *The Individual Psychology of Alfred Adler*. Harper & Row; 1956/1964.
3 Gilligan C. *In a Different Voice: psychological theory and women's development*. Harvard University Press; 1982.

to defend ourselves or our opinion; we are too compliant. We tend to operate through guile and passive-aggressive wheedling and manipulation instead of communicating cleanly and honestly.[4]

Gilligan feels this may be attributed to two types of thinking that differentiate the sexes: one based on concepts of rules, fairness and justice, and one based on feelings of compassion, care and concern for others.

This may be situational/social not physiological, but there is no doubt that woman are socialised to become highly sensitised to the needs of others: our default setting is non-confrontational; we avoid situations where we have to defend ourselves or our opinion. As professional working adults, despite being accomplished and driven, we are also compliant. To maintain this stance is anything but effortless. We may be high achieving, but our psychological profile lags behind our academic one. We sacrifice essential self-knowledge and self-expression to the pressure of who we think we ought to be.[5]

This is not to say that any of us women should give up our well-developed attributes of compassion and being empathetic, but that we can learn to understand why and what we feel, and begin to tolerate these emotions. Many men too, who are hard-wired differently, would benefit from learning how to develop skills of empathy, compassionate attention and good listening.

If you go on holiday, do you feel panicked by the amount of work left and return a day earlier to sort things out? If you do not tell a senior male clinician that he has made a mistake because it might impact badly, or find it difficult being a female managing men, or refuse offers of help because you feel you should be able to cope, or feel you are the only one with the skills to do it properly anyway, you are most likely a woman. You are denying your own needs and wishes at the expense of others. Women are brought up to have a sense of obligation to others. We make ourselves available to others to our own detriment, and, ultimately, to other's too. Our compassion traps us, which is why it is important to harness some assertiveness skills.

We all have needs, rights, opinions and choices that we have a right to exercise. Because of cultural pressures, women in particular find it difficult to acknowledge these needs and rights, and to own them. In the following section we explore some of the cultural conditioning that has led to an increased awareness of stereotypical gender-specific behaviours. It is important for us to explore this so that we can sharpen up our interpersonal and diagnostic skills and learn to 'read' those we communicate with better and so understand how best to communicate back. Remember too that we are discussing some broad gender stereotypes, not gender identity or sexuality – there is a whole spectrum of difference out there.

---

4   Simmonds R. *The Curse of the Good Girl*. Penguin Books; 2009.
5   Ibid.

Society and patriarchal culture has shaped all of us, and there are gender-specific roles and expectations that play out. Men and women clearly differ in their life experience, in their presentation and socialisation. The roles men and women play out have an impact on how they feel about themselves, their value and their role in the world. What do the roles say about our beliefs in ourselves, our outer versus inner worlds? A bigger role in the outer world makes us more assertive, more confident, and gives us higher self-esteem.

EXPLORING DIFFERENCE

If we spend some time exploring the inner world of mean and women, class and culture, we will see how sociological and physiological factors influence us. The following exercises are designed to help us think about these differences, and how patriarchal culture has shaped some of them. In considering some of the roles men and women play out in our society, there are still gender-specific roles and expectations that play out, although obviously looking back in time, the differences were more polarised.

EXERCISE 1

Think about the roles of women and men in your childhood, or your parent's childhood compared with now – what are the obvious changes? What are the stereotypical preferences in life roles at home, at work?

	Twentieth century	*Twenty-first century*
Men		
Women		
Boys		
Girls		

EXERCISE 2

How do men and women differ in their life experience, in their presentation, in their socialisation? What opportunities exist for both? Draw life-lines for different cultures and classes, poor and moneyed, and note the similarities and differences.

Birth	Old age
Birth	Old age
Birth	Old age

What are the current stereotypical preferences in life roles at home, at work? Think of yourself, your parents, people you know. Which would you attribute honestly to men and which to women. Who does the main bulk of the childcare? The school run? The housework? Who does what? Are certain roles gender-aligned? Who does the shopping, laundry, cleaning? The gardening, mending the car? Taking out the rubbish? Who takes the children out, or is this shared? Does anyone in your family care for an elderly parent? How was this role decided? Who has the most leisure time in your family: reading the paper, resting, pursuing hobbies? Who works where, in what role – part or full time? Who earns the most? Who spends the most time engaging with the world outside, and in what capacity: work or leisure? How would this look if it were charted? The roles men and women play out have an impact on how they feel about themselves, their value and their role in the world. What do the roles say about our beliefs in ourselves, our outer versus inner worlds? A bigger role in the outer world makes us more assertive, more confident, and gives us higher self-esteem.

EXERCISE 3

How did/do men and women behave differently with girl and boy babies – in their choice of clothes, games, toys, play? Generally, men's play with both girl and boy babies is more expansive, outward looking, physically challenging, rough and tumble. Women's play with their babies is more inward-focussed, more nurturing, more likely to teach socialisation and communication skills.

	Boys	*Girls*
Men		
Women		

EXERCISE 4

On a scale of 1 to 10, how socially confidant as a woman do you feel, at work or out and about? What confidence levels would you assume for men in similar situations? There is a very basic fear that operates in most oppressed groups – including women – around sexual harassment or assault – a vague threat of physical assault even if none intended/happens: male presence is threatening to women in situations where they feel vulnerable, walking home in the dark, for example. Likewise, some women feel uncomfortable in the presence of men using sexual innuendo and jokes.

Home: 1 .... 5 10

Work: 1 .... 5 10

Other: 1 .... 5 10

LINGUISTIC ASSUMPTIONS AND EXPECTATIONS

We know that gender and culture differences mean that things said one way are interpreted differently by others. There are differences in the way men and women vie for power, for status and for connection in their communication styles. If we explore some of these differences, and their impact on the ways men and women communicate, together and with each other, we can see how this affects our ability to be assertive.

Language enables us to communicate in many different ways, for many different purposes. We do not always mean what we say.[6] When we say 'yes',

---

6   Townsend J. Paralinguistics: it's not what you say it's the way that you say it. *Management Decision*. 1988; **26**(3): 26–40. Crystal D. Prosody and paralinguistic correlates of social categories. In: Gardener E, editor. *Social Anthropology and Language*. Tavistock Press; 1971. pp. 185–206.

we do not always mean it: politeness dictates our inability to say 'no'. We can speak the same word or sentence with altogether different meaning, with the meaning conveyed in the tone (of voice), the stress, pausing, intonation and context. The way the sentence is phrased, the syntax – word order – will also have an impact.

Argyle[7] was one of the first psychologists to put forward the hypothesis that whereas spoken language is normally used for communicating information about events external to the speakers, non-verbal codes are used to establish and maintain interpersonal relationships. Paralinguistics is the term used for the study of how things are said and how this affects the meaning of what is said: it looks at language purposes, some of the hidden meanings, expectations and assumptions in our language, some of the ways we communicate, and includes the study of how men and women's discourse differs.

Beneath language there are always hidden meanings. There is an unstated but 'heard' hierarchical ranking/power dynamic that plays out. We are aware that a GP, for example, will almost always be respectfully called 'doctor' by their patient, whereas a health visitor, midwife or therapist will be called, more informally, by their first name. Rank is insidious and crucial. Compliments are almost always given by those of higher rank to those of lower rank, and talk/subject matter is always initiated by the higher ranking. This ranking means that unspoken rules are followed, there are hidden expectations and assumptions in the meaning behind the language. Thus, if a person of higher 'rank' asks 'You don't mind if I do X do you?', there is an expectation that the person of lower rank will accede. The implied meaning behind the statement is 'I am being polite but my expectation is that you will agree with me': the expectation is thwarted if the answer is 'no'; the refusal becomes challenging.

Both genders have different repertoires and we have different expectations about how men and women present, their expectations, their core beliefs. This affects the way people, the public, our patients/clients, managers, view us, so it is important to acknowledge. Deborah Tannen[8] is one of the biggest researchers into language discourse and gender. She demonstrates how, for example, men and women, girls and boys, differ in their use of 'air time', the type of vocabulary used, levels of directness, how they may interrupt as a device to dominate (or to indicate desperation), how they use silence versus volubility to indicate status or connection. Her work shows how women tend towards connection and sharing; men towards hierarchy, problem solving and building status.

---

7   Argyle M, Salter V, Nicholson H, *et al.* The communication of inferior and superior attitudes by verbal and non-verbal signals. *British Journal of Social and Clinical Psychology.* 1970; 9: 222–31.
8   Tannen D. *You Just Don't Understand: women and men in conversation.* Virago Press; 1992. Tannen D. *Talking from 9 to 5: women and men at work: language, sex and power.* Virago Press; 1996.

Her work shows that in conflict, women are more likely to withdraw, whereas men more happily meet conflict with verbal aggression. Women do use more words, and as a rule have a larger vocabulary, and use it! We differ too in our use of questioning – men tend to use questions much more pragmatically, to gain information; they use more 'closed' questions that require a one word or yes/no response. Women use 'open' questioning more to expand the conversation and elicit more feeling/emotional understanding about the topic ('How?', 'Why did it happen?'). Women tend to ask questions to help them understand the other person. Men feel more comfortable staying on topic, with conversation following a more direct, linear, 'spotlight' path, whereas women can be happier meandering off topic, chatting for the sake of continuing an emotional connection. Men often have the confidence to interrupt, but are more likely to interrupt someone of lower rank, women included. They are more likely to use expressions of conflict and verbal aggression, to raise topics of interest to themselves and to behave with high confidence. Women have some known conversational rituals, with more frequent apology. Thus there is a hidden agenda in any discourse, where conversation plays out hidden issues of patriarchy, power and solidarity.

There are differences in the type of vocabulary used too. Women have some known conversational rituals, with more frequent apology; and men are more assertive generally. In male discourse, men are much more likely than women to use sporting or defence metaphors 'stick to your guns/ballpark figure/an uphill battle/it's in the can', for example.

There are different expectations too about how men and women present, their expectations, their core beliefs. What follows are some commonly used female discourse patterns. It is worth considering the circumstances when women switch discourses. Women use different registers and communication styles depending on the circumstances: we are much more likely to switch our communication style when circumstances dictate and contexts change – if at work, home, socialising; whether we aim to flatter or console, impress or indicate submission.

Female discourse patterns:

➤ to believe, and say, they have got it wrong
➤ indirectness
➤ happy with silence
➤ raising topics of interest to listener
➤ low confidence/aggression
➤ frequent apologies
➤ asking lots of questions to gain information and understand the other person
➤ more likely to adapt to the style of speaker
➤ waiting for turn to come before speaking

- ➤ smiling more
- ➤ non-verbal attentiveness ('silent applause'): listening, observing, quiet, sympathetic approach
- ➤ more deferential, keeping quiet about their successes
- ➤ asking men what interests them and listening
- ➤ better at reciprocal communication, keeping the flow going between both parties, taking turns
- ➤ communicating with less certainty and confidence, diffident but with more respect for feelings: 'This might seem a silly question but …', 'You've probably thought of this before, but …'
- ➤ apologising, taking blame, admitting ignorance
- ➤ using an attenuated/personal voice: 'I'm intrigued by your comment, can you say a bit more?'
- ➤ more likely to back off if interrupted, less likely to persist
- ➤ building on others questions, asking questions to elicit ideas
- ➤ tentative communication: speaking with low confidence/aggression: no boasting/bragging, downplaying their own authority
- ➤ seeking agreement before changing topics: '… shall we look at X now?'
- ➤ avoiding stating they have revised/planned activity/schedule – feeling discomfort with power
- ➤ agreeing, supporting, encouraging: making suggestions not commanding
- ➤ more likely to adapt to the style of speaker
- ➤ waiting for turn to come before speaking.

It is thought by psychologists[9] that at about 12 years old, girls disconnect from their full range of feelings in order to fit in and garner the good opinion of others. There is even a physiological component to this: when a girl is ready to be 'good', her voice rises. This simple outward change is one of the changes that is indicative of a girl giving up her full range of feelings and rendering herself selfless.

To counteract this, assertive messages can be conveyed both verbally and non-verbally, and part of being assertive is knowing how to conduct yourself with maturity and confidence using the appropriate posture, gesture, vocal pitch and facial expressions. This is not a question of acting. You need to *feel* assertive, not just to behave as though you are, otherwise a covert message leaks out. It is difficult to disguise powerful emotions as body language reveals true feelings. It is possible, though, to build your confidence and self-esteem simply by adjusting your posture or appearance, or even your vocal range. You will

---

9   Mikel Brown L, Gilligan C. *Meeting at the Crossroads: women's psychology and girls' development.* Harvard University Press; 1992. Mozzarella S, Pecora N. Revisiting girl's studies. *Journal of Children and Media.* 2007; **1**(2): 105–25.

show more authority if you stand face to face with someone, rather than if you sit and they stand, and if you lower the pitch of your voice and slightly increase the volume.

When considering the default female qualities, it is harder to give a firm and clear 'no' when you have been socialised to be more compliant, to apologise, to have lower confidence in yourself and your abilities and rights. As a woman, one way you can regain some power, and learn to stand up for yourself and your needs, is to take a critical look at how you present as a woman. Does your presentation and body language 'mark' you as someone without much power and authority? If you are unhappy with this, make a conscious decision to present yourself more strongly. Check your body language: make sure you look the person in the eye as you say 'no', or try moving away or making a 'no' hand movement. Check that you are not smiling apologetically as you talk, maintain firm eye contact, sit or stand upright, and keep your voice steady and clear.

To help in this process, start to unpick what you see about yourself compared with how others present themselves. Look for signs of dominance and submission in people's verbal and non-verbal behaviour, looking at both 'gross' and 'fine' features: large body movements, sitting, standing, arm crossing; eye movements, facial expressions, tone of voice, etc.

EXERCISE 5

Begin to watch people. Compare video/radio footage/observe them on public transport. Soaps and dramas make excellent observation platforms, because the behaviours are so extreme and stereotypical. Make a rough count of your observations. Make a mental note of the behaviours you see on a continuum of submissive/passive and confident/aggressive. Who crosses their legs, smiles most frequently? Who takes up the seats on public transport, unapologetically? Who stares, who challenges? The verbal and non-verbal features to observe are as follows.

Gross:
➤ body space
➤ body positioning
➤ facial expressions
➤ head positioning – head tilt, clear listening behaviour
➤ emotional literacy: ability to understand emotions from facial expression.

Fine (verbal communication/suprasegmentals):
➤ pitch
➤ vocal tone
➤ accuracy of articulation
➤ resonance

➤ breathiness/quality
➤ vocal inflections.

EXERCISE 6

Map who takes up the most verbal space when men and women are together. In which situations (compare meetings at work with those in the pub)?

	Body space/ dominance	Use of gesture	Facial expressions	'Air time'
Men				
Women				

As a general rule, observe that men tend towards taking up more space physically, with less apology. They tend to show less facial expression. (It has been suggested that with men it is important to maintain the hierarchy, to keep their feelings intact and hidden,[10] to protect against another man 'gaining' knowledge about them. Thus they are often less able or willing to understand emotions from facial expression.)

BECOMING ASSERTIVE

Body language

Patriarchy puts women and children in a subservient space – this can be corrected by taking up as much space as men. From previous exercises, you may have observed how, in public and private spaces, a man confident of their position and power opens their body up – they may sprawl their legs, arms behind their head, akimbo. They may place their possessions (briefcase, etc.) in an extended space beside them to increase their territorial range. Their voices are stronger and carry further (listen to the mobile phone users). Women do not permit themselves this privilege; their clothing is often restrictive, forcing the body to close in, restricting the space taken up and limiting the power base. We may not feel comfortable or need to adopt men's dress or postures – but we can redress the balance by taking equal space ourselves, in our own way.

---

10 Tannen (1992, 1996), note 8 above.

Posture and distance

Assertive behaviour:

➤ stand or sit upright and relaxed, with your feet firmly on the ground

➤ deepen your breathing and calm yourself

➤ check to see if you are too near the other person, which can be construed as confrontational

➤ whoever sits or stands in a higher position is the dominant one – raise or lower your chair to meet the other as an equal

➤ be still, and use open hand movements

➤ avoid a timid, tentative walk – enter a room as if you belong there

➤ do not smile too much; do not smile at all if it is not in keeping with the seriousness of what you are saying

➤ maintain eye contact by looking at the other person in a relaxed, friendly, confident way.

Watch out for:

➤ impatience, indicated through striding, leaning over or finger pointing

➤ dominant or aggressive behaviour – use of too much space, crossing arms to indicate inapproachability or protection

➤ nervous twiddling, clasping and unclasping of the hands or shuffling feet

➤ tapping or chopping hand movements, which are construed to be aggressive and impatient

➤ covering your mouth with your hand

➤ smiling inappropriately – women often smile involuntarily when angry or critical (as we have been socialised to deal with angry feeling indirectly and do not feel comfortable conveying them clearly)

➤ staring, which is intimidating – the intimidated person evades eye contact or looks down, the nervous looks away.

Facial expressions and intonation

Our voice is very important to us in many ways. What happens to your voice when you speak with someone on the telephone; what can you tell about them from their voice? What happens when you feel pleased and happy to see someone, or you are angry? Think of someone whose voice is easy to listen to. What qualities does their voice have? Women tend towards more obvious changes in pitch, vocal tone and inflection. They have better accuracy of articulation (clinical observation shows they are less likely to mumble, omit word endings, use glottal stops). Women have better developed non-verbal communication skills.

Which of the following traits are preferable to listen to?

loud/soft	fast rate/slow	clear/imprecise enunciation
high/low pitch	tuneful/monotonous	

Thinking of these traits, try reading a passage, altering your voice. How do you sound? The following voice features are very much interlinked: slow speech = more precise speech; raised pitch = louder voice. If you relax and breath deeply, using diaphragmatic not chest breathing, your voice will be clearer and resonate well. Keep your voice steady and fluent, neither too loud nor too soft, and lower it a fraction. The assertive speaker avoids whining, shouting or conveying sarcasm; aggressive speech – clipped, fast and abrupt; and over-soft, quiet, trailing off speaking patterns. The passive person speaks quietly and hesitantly with frequent pausing.

EXERCISE 7

Ask a friend to rate your voice:

Pitch	1 5	....	10
Volume	1 5	....	10
Speed	1 5	....	10
Assertiveness rating	1 5	....	10

Then role play. Using the situations as a guide, apply some of the above principles and think about your use of power/authority, body language, choice of words and ways of saying things (softly, calmly, kindly, etc.)

➤ giving someone feedback on their work (at work)
➤ a colleague at work asks you a challenging question (does your approach differ when the member of staff is male or female?)
➤ your manager disciplines you for forgetting to complete an important piece of work.

EXERCISE 8

Understanding non–verbal behaviour

In the following exercise, think about:

➤ eye contact
➤ seating positions
➤ loudness of voice

➤ tone of voice
➤ facial expression
➤ body posture.

Choose a neutral sentence ('Great to see you'; 'When is your birthday?'). Using the same sentence, convey the following emotions to a partner. Can they guess the emotion? What leads them to think as they do?

- Openness.
- Defensive.
- Evaluating.
- Suspiciously.
- With readiness.
- Insecurely.
- Co-operatively.

- Excited.
- Puzzled.
- Frightened.
- Interested.
- Irritated.
- Depressed.
- Anxious.

- Surprised.
- Sarcastic.
- Critical.
- Bored.
- Frightened.

DEVELOPING AN IMAGE

A professional image

Take an honest look at how you present: the more feminine your image, the more female your presentation, the less seriously you will be taken professionally. If you feel this is the case, and if you want to, tone it down a fraction, remembering that within your choice of image it is still possible to show strength of character and keep your power with words and body language. Think seriously about what your appearance says about the impression you wish to convey to others. Look at other colleagues. What is it about them that suggests authority? There is an unspoken NHS dress code, backed up by policy: take time to look critically at what each look conveys. Authority or seniority is usually understated, with clothing simple and formal. Aim for a personal style to express your own individuality. Dress codes may be relaxing in the workplace, but this may not obviate your need to boost your self-esteem by dressing in a particular way. Dress in a way that genuinely makes you feel comfortable and efficient. Many women do not reflect the importance of their jobs in the way they look or act. Their style lags behind their titles.

Self-publicise to build your confidence

Men find it easier than women to self-publicise. Women are not socialised to 'show off'. But, especially at work, people will not see you as important unless you project that importance: they forget your accomplishments if you do not keep them informed.

➤ Recognise your achievements and take credit for them; do not assume your accomplishments are routine.

➤ Let other people's opinions of you do the talking, as in, 'I was asked to make the key speech at the conference this year' or 'I'll be tied up next week: I'm heading the new clinical governance project'.

➤ Angle your stories to highlight any assertive qualities: 'I negotiated my way through that situation, and we both achieved outcomes we were happy with.'

Here you are implementing a carefully calculated reporting system designed to let people know what you are doing – so that they will give you the opportunity to do more. Remember that confidence and high self-esteem are indicated when you no longer need to conform to someone else's standard, so find your own style, which may be to be quieter and less assuming, but ruthlessly efficient.

Non-assertive people spend a considerable amount of time understanding, acknowledging and fulfilling other people's needs. They fear disapproval because it threatens their sense of self-esteem; they want to be liked, so avoid standing up for themselves. Assertive people successfully assess their own behaviour, release themselves from dependence on the opinions of others, accept their own vulnerabilities and inherent desire to be liked. They choose for themselves, freeing themselves from manipulative behaviour and resentments.

Even today, many men have only known women as subordinates. No matter how knowledgeable and skilled, female clinicians and managers may still be perceived as flirtatious, competitive, too warm or too hard. Some men feel a loss of identity; they feel invaded, insecure and threatened by competent women. These men need to be educated to become better 'process' observers. They fail to perceive emotional cues and need to learn to respond with understanding in the same way. Women can assist by continuous determination for a professional relationship – mutual help, information-sharing and socialisation. As we model good professional and management behaviour, we break down prejudices and help men form new expectations of us.

Women's advantage is our well-developed communication skills – we are more able at developing and maintaining communication links, more capable of building reciprocal relationships of great potential and mutual benefit, very good at process observation, trained to pick up other's discomforts, anxieties, fears and angers, and able to respond to emotions instinctively. An impressive list, and one that lends us to learning to be more assertive. However, because of these skills, women also often say much more about the way they feel than they then feel comfortable with.

We need to remember that we too are intelligent, capable and equal human beings, especially when we feel undermined by our imperialist medical system that assumes medics, and men in particular, hold the power. Health and social care are hierarchical organisations with unwritten rules at play. The medics and those in senior positions dominate the hierarchy, which leaves women managers in particular in a much less powerful position. In many workplaces information is withheld (only certain people are allowed access to the medical notes/information/meetings); doctors may be cynical, disenchanted, defensive and obstructive of change (and only the doctors are permitted to prescribe, judge, decide, diagnose); and managers have to fight their way through the system to be heard.

Medicine is still often practised in an anachronistic, parochial and patriarchal way, with the balance of power held by the medics. Only recently, the press reported a newly retired consultant as saying, under the banner heading 'Cut surplus NHS chiefs':

> 'Doctors and nurses are under threat of being fired or having their contracts negotiated, while chief executives direct operations on inflated salaries. Some of them earn more than the highest paid consultants in the NHS … for years it has been apparent to us that enormous sums can be saved by cutting bureaucracy and management costs in the NHS. A hospital can run its own affairs with a medical superintendent, matron and administrator. This was how it was done before modern management was thrust upon us.'[11]

This type of comment, not unusual, shows an extraordinary arrogance, insensitivity and lack of knowledge of the hard work of their colleagues, and unparalleled misunderstanding of the cost and operations in running a multi-million pound healthcare business.

This is shifting as those in less powerful positions are gaining more confidence and authority to question the medical ascendancy model. People become more assertive as they become more informed. They demand information and value for money, and are not so easily placated. Women in healthcare therefore need to grow into the skills demanded of them, develop their confidence and become more assertive. The first step is to build self-esteem, belief in your own abilities, and reduce self-blame.

If you always reproach yourself when things go wrong, especially when the fault does not lie with you, you need to put the blame where it belongs. If we have grown up with over-critical caregivers, we realise that we have broken the regulations only when we get punished. As a result, we develop a sensitive spot, an alarm that signals we are at fault, a sense of responsibility that is usefully triggered when we genuinely make mistakes. Less usefully, this alarm also goes off as an advance warning when a mistake has been made and it is not clear whose error it is. In response to that guilty inner flinch, we quickly respond to offload the discomfort by blaming someone else, or take the blame ourselves.

---

11 Evans H, Evans S (retired consultant surgeon and retired nurse). Cut surplus NHS chiefs [letter]. *The Sunday Times*. 2012 Jul 22.

Research shows that while men look outside themselves to see why things have gone wrong, women look inside and blame themselves.[12] Accepting fault feels more comfortable. It avoids conflict, nurtures others and smoothes over relationships. This can be challenged by acting in a positive, constructive way: register that in some way you could have done better and that you will take better action next time. Taking blame means buying into the belief that all errors are your fault. The hopelessness and negativity are destructive and do nothing to help you deal with the problem. Challenge any negative self-talk (nobody is perfect) with something more constructive: ' I know how to do this well, it is only fear that is making it difficult.' Look to yourself more compassionately. If fear is blocking your assertive responses, try these guidelines. These are especially useful if you are working with clients to build their self-esteem.

1   Accept responsibility, not blame

➤ Spot the physical warning signs: your stomach churning, or a voice in your head saying: 'It's my fault again.'
➤ Note your automatic apology and offer to put things right.
➤ Assess whether this is an appropriate response.
➤ If it is not, stop, reflect and start to break the pattern.

2   Challenge your accusers

When someone who blames you, what they are actually doing is offloading their own discomfort. Men and children, in particular, will routinely shift responsibility to external circumstances – and that means you. So 'Where's my laptop?' becomes 'Where did you put my laptop?'. The implication is clear. If people threaten you, 'You said you would make this work!', you could try to open out the choices: 'I said I would try and make it work, we have a joint responsibility here to make this happen ...'

3   Quick ways to reduce the blame

➤ Wait. Listen to the other person (or the self-blame you are putting on yourself) rather than rushing in, without thinking, to apologise or explain.
➤ Relax: feeling physically better will make you emotionally more resilient.
➤ Check the messages you are sending out. Stand relaxed and easy, keep eye contact rather than looking away defensively.

4   Convert blame into action

➤ Sort out the problem that created the blame in the first place.
➤ Focus on what positive action you can take.

---

12 Tannen (1992, 1996), note 8 above. Dickson A. *The Mirror Within: a new look at sexuality.* Quartet Books; 1985.

➤ do things on my own
➤ look good
➤ feel physically fit
➤ like myself
➤ achieve things
➤ give affection
➤ be respected?

Which needs are most, and least, satisfied? What can you do towards satisfying your least satisfied needs?

In summary, we have seen that women are expected by society to be more compliant than challenging and more obedient than ambitious. Other qualities, like leadership, taking full responsibility for the outcome of things and risk-taking, are not encouraged. But these are the very things required of us in the world of work. It is hoped this chapter has helped to begin to explain the position of women in society and why we have to work so much harder than men at being assertive, and given some ideas about the best way to challenge some of our habitual patterns of behaviour. It is time to move forward and begin to take charge of our lives.

KEY POINTS

➤ There are gender-specific roles and expectations that play out in our society. Men and women differ in their life experience, in their presentation and socialisation: different opportunities exist for each.
➤ Assertiveness is particularly important for women. In terms of assertiveness, we look at patriarchy and feminism to explain the sense of inferiority that women have. Personal, political and cultural approaches are needed to understand why we behave as we do.
➤ Woman are socialised to become highly sensitised to the needs of others; our default setting is non-confrontational. Our compassion traps us.
➤ Men generally find it easier to be assertive, but some find it harder to develop the fine-tuned and complex verbal and non-verbal skills needed to listen and communicate with empathy, sympathy and focus.
➤ Although patriarchy puts men in the stronger position, they are facing a confusing and transforming time, under pressure to reconstruct their masculinity in the face of an increasingly feminised society.
➤ Paralinguistics looks at language purposes, some of the hidden meanings, expectations and assumptions in our language, some of the ways we communicate, and includes the study of how men and women's discourse differs.

➤ Language enables us to communicate in many different ways, for many different purposes. The way a sentence is phrased, the syntax – word order – will also have an impact. Gender and culture differences mean that things said one way are interpreted differently by others. There are differences in the way men and women vie for power, for status and for connection in their communication styles.

➤ You need to *feel* assertive, not just behave as though you are, otherwise a covert message leaks out. It is difficult to disguise powerful emotions as body language reveals true feelings.

➤ As women model good professional and management behaviour, we break down prejudices and help men to form new expectations of us.

➤ The health service is still a hierarchical organisation with unwritten rules at play. This is shifting: those in less powerful positions are gaining more confidence and authority to question the medical ascendancy model.

➤ Work blocks for women: we can be too honest, are too nice, we need to learn to develop a sense of strategy and see socialising as an important part of work. We need to begin to look like women who take complete responsibility for themselves.

➤ We need to recognise the value of competition, accept responsibility, challenge our accusers, convert blame into action, live by our own standards, and choose when to apologise. We may take on certain beliefs about ourselves because we feel powerless to reject them, but it is possible to reconsider and change them.

FURTHER READING

Back K, Back K. *Assertiveness at Work: a practical guide to handling awkward situations.* 3rd ed. McGraw-Hill Professional; 2005.

Jeffers S. *Feel the Fear and Do it Anyway: how to turn your fear and indecision into confidence and action.* 20th anniversary ed. Vermilion; 2007.

Jeffers S. *The Little Book of Confidence.* Rider Books; 1999.

Speer SA. *Gender Talk. Feminism, discourse and conversation analysis.* Routledge; 2005.

Swiss D. *The Male Mind at Work: a woman's guide to working with men.* Basic Books; 2001.

CHAPTER 3

How to be assertive

The *Oxford English Dictionary* definition of assertive is:

> 'Having or showing a confident and forceful personality e.g.: patients should be more assertive with their doctors.'

The *Dorland's Medical Dictionary* definition is fuller:

> 'Assertiveness: a form of behaviour characterized by a confident declaration or affirmation of a statement without need of proof; this affirms the person's rights or point of view without either aggressively threatening the rights of another (assuming a position of dominance) or submissively permitting another to ignore or deny one's rights or point of view.'

The first definition describes the commonly held view of assertiveness; the second lies closer to the truth of what we currently teach.

The following chapters point you in the direction of the skills you need to learn to become assertive. Although some of these may look simple, as with making any behavioural change, you will need to practise regularly, challenge yourself and move out of your comfort zone fully to develop a fluid ability and expertise. We all have our own preferred communication styles, and in learning how to become assertive some of these habitual ways of communicating and being will be changed or modified, and this needs courage, determination and practice.

EARLY DEVELOPMENTS

Assertiveness is increasingly singled out as a behavioural skill taught by many personal development experts, psychological and cognitive behavioural therapists. During the second half of the twentieth century, the term and concept was popularised to the general public through books and training courses, and this continues today.

To gain some understanding of the level of individual change required to become more assertive, we need to look to the early school of work developed by cognitive therapists. Cognitive therapy is a type of psychotherapy first developed by an American psychiatrist, Aaron Beck.[1] It is one of the therapeutic approaches within the larger group of cognitive behaviour therapies and was first expounded by Beck in the 1960s.

Cognitive therapy seeks to help people overcome difficulties by identifying and changing dysfunctional thinking, behaviour and emotional responses. This involves helping to develop skills for modifying beliefs, identifying distorted thinking, relating to others in different ways and changing behaviours. The work is based on testing beliefs and assumptions and identifying how some of our usually unquestioned thoughts are distorted, unrealistic and unhelpful. Once those thoughts have been challenged, our feelings about the subject matter (of those thoughts) are more easily subject to change. Beck initially focused on working with depression and raising self-esteem. He developed a list of 'errors', faulty thinking that he proposed could maintain depression, including over-generalisation, magnification of negatives and minimisation of positives. He also introduced a focus on the underlying 'schema' – the fundamental underlying ways in which people process information – about the self, the world or the future.

In working with behavioural change, such as learning assertiveness skills, we need to address the way we think and behave in response to situations and develop more flexible ways to think and respond, including reducing the avoidance of activities. Beck's work was predicated on his disillusion with long-term psychodynamic approaches based on gaining insight into unconscious emotions and drives. He came to the conclusion that the way in which his clients perceived, interpreted and attributed meaning in their daily lives was key to cognitive change.[2] At the same time, he was working on similar ideas from a different perspective, in developing his rational emotive behaviour therapy. Both approaches were fundamental in the early stages of work on assertiveness, but a more modern approach does now incorporate some personal awareness work, through making the unconscious more conscious.

In the 1970s, there was a cognitive revolution in psychology. Behavioural modification techniques and cognitive therapy techniques became joined together, giving rise to the cognitive behaviour therapy we know today.

So, to become assertive one has to notice and overcome difficulties by identifying and changing dysfunctional thinking, behaviour and emotional responses. This will involve developing skills for modifying beliefs, identifying

---

1 Beck JS, Beck AT. *Cognitive Behavior Therapy: basics and beyond* [hardcover]. 2nd ed. The Guilford Press; 2011. Beck AT. The current state of cognitive therapy: a 40-year retrospective. *Arch Gen Psychiatry*. 2005; **62**(9): 953–9.

2 Beck JS. *About Cognitive Therapy*. Beck Institute for Cognitive Therapy and Research; 1979 (retrieved 21 November 2008). Beck AT, Rush AJ, Shaw BF, *et al. Cognitive Therapy of Depression*. The Guilford Press; 1979.

distorted thinking, relating to others in different ways and changing behaviours. You will need to gain awareness of and test your beliefs and assumptions about yourself and your world, and identify how some of your usually unquestioned thoughts and behaviours are distorted or dysfunctional, unrealistic or unhelpful. Once those thoughts have been challenged, your feelings and your behaviours have a chance to change.

HOW TO BE ASSERTIVE

Assertive communication is honest and direct; it is speaking your mind without fudging the issue or being aggressive. The assertive speaker is prepared to:
➤ be specific
➤ be honest and open
➤ negotiate
➤ repeat their message if misunderstood
➤ compromise if it is reasonable to do so
➤ listen
➤ self-disclose – express their feelings
➤ innovate – take chances and risks
➤ accept criticism where appropriate
➤ prompt others to express themselves honestly.

We know we are assertive people when we have the following characteristics.
➤ We feel free to express our feelings, thoughts, and desires.
➤ We are able to initiate and maintain comfortable relationships with others.
➤ We know our rights.
➤ We have control over our anger. This does not mean that we repress this feeling; it means that we control anger and talk about it in a reasoning manner.
➤ We are willing to compromise with others.
➤ We tend to have good self-esteem.
➤ We connect with others with mutual respect, acknowledging we both have needs, and although these might be different, they are no more or less.

Assertive communication usually leaves both speaker and listener feeling more comfortable than avoidance or confrontation.

In order to behave assertively, we need to take more personal responsibility for ourselves. Scott Peck, a psychologist, noted that our behaviour is often motivated by trying to appoint someone else – a manager, partner, friend – to be responsible for our problems.[3] To reduce any possible

---

3 Peck MS. *The Road Less Travelled*. Arrow; 1990.

pain of taking responsibility, we give away our power. This makes sense in childhood, but if it persists into adulthood it breeds resentment and pain. The entirety of our adult life is spent making personal decisions and choices. If we accept this, then we are free and empowered to accept any consequences of our decisions.

We also need to protect and take care of ourselves by setting personal boundaries. We need to be able to tell other people when they are acting in ways that are not acceptable to us. A first step is starting to know that we have a right to protect and defend ourselves. Perhaps we have not only the right, but also the adult duty to take responsibility for how we allow others to treat us. One way to do this is to acknowledge and understand our own feelings, to 'own' our own voice and the right to speak up for our selves. It is impossible to have a good, healthy relationship with someone who has no boundaries, with someone who cannot communicate directly and honestly. Learning how to set boundaries is a necessary step in learning to be a friend to ourselves. It is our responsibility to take care of ourselves – to protect ourselves when it is necessary. It is impossible to learn to take care of ourselves without owning our own feelings and the rights and responsibilities as co-creators of our lives.

Many working in healthcare are already skilled communicators, as they are selected for, or trained in, interpersonal communication skills. However, we all have black spots, so it is worth reflecting on some of your own skills.

Step 1: Understand yourself

In order to recognise assertiveness in yourself, question if there is a pattern in the way you interact with people, and remember the times when something you did or said worked well. It is likely if the communication went well, one of you was being assertive.

Use the following exercises to begin to understand yourself, to find out how you are likely to respond in a given situation, with whom, under which circumstances. If you are interested in understanding more about how and why you, or others, behave in a certain way in more detail, *see* Section 4.

EXERCISE 1

Write a list of five situations in which you would like to behave more assertively, with open, direct and honest communication.

> Then next to each situation, note your current response:
>
> **P = passive, A = aggressive or I = indirect (manipulative)**

EXERCISE 2

For each of the scenarios below, ask yourself the following.

➤ What did you feel?

➤ Was your response aggressive, passive, assertive or manipulative?

➤ Were you aware of any non-verbal behaviours demonstrated?

➤ What would you see as an alternative, assertive response?

1 A member of staff gives a blank 'no' when you make a request for them to attend training.

2 A colleague interrupts your work, asking you to show an unexpected visitor round because they are unable to as their meeting/clinic/surgery is just beginning.

3 Your manager or one of the partners suddenly accuses you of attending too many meetings away from the practice/office – you are never available when needed. Is this a fair or unfair criticism?

4 A member of staff accuses you of talking behind their back about them. Is this a fair or unfair criticism?

EXERCISE 3

➤ List *who*, in friendships, work or family, makes you feel either passive or aggressive.

➤ List *when* you have behaved non-assertively.

➤ List *what* subjects make you feel, and behave, non-assertively, for example, when making mistakes, discussing politics or expressing negative feelings.

Step 2: The basics of assertive behaviour

Here we look at some of the basic skills of assertiveness, the skills that are relatively easy to learn and which we can begin to use daily in situations that are not too challenging, provocative or difficult. The checklists below give a favour of a style of communicating more honestly and directly. This leaves both parties feeling clearer and more comfortable with the interaction. The following ways of communicating help the most in difficult or problematic situations – when dealing with critical comments or manipulative behaviour, having to give criticism, or when negotiating. It is very hard to change ingrained habits of behaviour, so a general rule is to pause and think before you speak, prepare/rehearse your speech with sympathetic friends or colleagues, and remember if the situation is problematic or awkward for then you are more likely to hesitate, digress, make mistakes. We can only learn from the mistakes, so have a go!

1   Be clear and specific

➤ Make the statement brief, and avoid unnecessary padding, especially when saying 'no' – 'sorry' and 'but' dilute the clarity and expose your uncertainty.
➤ Own your statement, assume responsibility.
➤ Keep your statement simple, brief and direct.

Example:

> 'I have noticed that you have been late to work on several occasions over the last month, Paula; I want to support you if you are having any difficulties: tell me about why this is.'

Do not pass the buck: this diminishes your credibility and marks you as someone who is not willing to address the issue firmly.

If you feel you are being criticised but the criticism is messy, manipulative and nebulous, seek clarity yourself. No one likes giving criticism, so it is often done badly:

> 'I'm not sure if you really enjoy the organisational side of your job … but the receptionists seem to like you.'

If the next kind of comment is directed at you, ask for clarity, take charge:

> 'Last time we met you said you were unsure I liked the organisational side of my work. What makes you think that?'

followed by something proactive about your own willingness to change:

> 'I'd like to look at some ways I can try and change this: do you have any ideas?'

Ask for clarification, and examples, to expose the criticism. This allows both parties to identify the issue and begin to tackle it. Clarity untangles unexpressed needs, manipulation, sarcasm, sulking. When you express a willingness to both accept the situation and look at changing it, you regain the power. For example:

Sagarika has, on the whole, a good relationship with her manager, but occasionally she leaves an encounter feeling belittled and uncomfortable. She is vaguely aware that she is being manipulated, and often feels criticised, but is finding it difficult to pinpoint. At the next meeting with her manager, she listens carefully to what is said, and finds that she is being subtly patronised. Having identified this, she is able to discuss her feelings with her manager.

Do not confuse clarity and directness with bluntness or rudeness. Being clear about an issue is being simple and intelligible about it. Being direct avoids the wish to whinge or complain, to respond in a roundabout way, or to reproach. If you are irritated by someone's untidiness, tell them what you are unhappy about. Unless you tell them, they will not know: they will not necessarily be able to see through your indirect sulks, nor may they correctly interpret them. Pinpoint the behaviour when it occurs. Ask for clarification or 'read' behind the statement. Be clear in your own mind first what the issue is that you want to tackle.

2   *Be open and honest about your feelings*
➤ Tell how you feel, own it.
➤ Do not hide behind words.
➤ Do not use words to manipulate or hurt.
➤ Never say 'You make me feel' – no one can make us feel anything, we take personal responsibility for our own feelings.
➤ Begin difficult situations with simple statements: 'I feel nervous/guilty/ angry …'

As we are rarely given the opportunity to explore negative feelings, this skill takes practise. To begin with, you may wish to notice the impact of your feelings physically, in your body, for example, a sinking feeling, a lump in the throat, a tight chest, sickness. Name these, and then eventually you will feel more able to respond honestly and quickly.

3   *Repeat your message*
This technique is sometimes called the 'stuck record' or 'broken record' technique. If you feel misunderstood, or need to diffuse anger, calmly repeat your statement or request. By such gentle persistence you can maintain your position without falling prey to manipulative comment, irrelevant logic or argumentative bait. This is an especially useful skill to use when dealing with aggressive people.
➤ Listen carefully to the other person's point of view.
➤ Acknowledge it.
➤ Then stick to your desired point.
➤ Repeat several times if necessary:

This will help you to ignore the verbal traps that people sometimes set to draw us in.

> 'I understand that you are feeling angry about the lack of appointments Mr Habib; this is something we are looking at and hoping to redress in the near future. I have logged your complaint.'

After hearing this three or four times, the complainant gets the message. On the telephone, and as a last resort, try saying cheerfully and politely 'Thank you for calling!' before putting the phone down. This firmly closes the conversation.

This technique is best used in situations when your time and energy is precious, or when your rights are in danger of being abused. It is particularly useful when seeking a refund for faulty goods, or when you are refusing someone something and they persist. Be clear that you are not going to give way. In the following example, a practice manager has just begun writing the second of a backlog of a dozen reports when one of the partners asks her to break off and see a drugs representative.

Example A

> Dr: 'Oh, good, here you are. Here is Abdul, from Bayer's. He has some information on a new product I'm interested in, and I'm in the middle of surgery. Can you have a word?'
>
> Manager: 'I'm sorry I can't help right now – I've just started working on these reports. Come in so we can make another appointment.'
>
> Dr: 'But this product is important – it represents big savings to the practice, can't you spare a little time?' [*manipulative bait – a plea to the manager's guilt*]
>
> Manager: 'No, I wish I had the time.' [*repeats*] 'I have a deadline to meet. Let's make it next Tuesday or Wednesday? I'd really like to hear about the product.'
>
> Dr: [*critically*] 'It won't take long, you know' [*irrelevant logic*].
>
> Manager: 'I understand its frustrating for both of you,' [*fielding the response and accepting some responsibility for the manipulative criticism*] 'but I really need to finish this now.'

The doctor finally accepts his manager's refusal, and respects her determination and ability to set her own priorities. The manager has not been led by the doctor's own inability to manage his time, or his aim to control her agenda. This classic situation is one where you are likely to be diverted by clever and articulate argument. Stay with what you need, relax and keep to your word. You may wish to alter the wording slightly each time, to avoid sounding artificial.

Example B

Lianne, a GP registrar who has just completed a dermatology placement, is in her office and is already late for a home visit, after which an important meeting is scheduled. She is packing her bags when Dr M, senior partner, knocks on the door in a fluster.

> Dr M: 'Oh, Good, you've not yet left for visits. Can you come and see Mr Jones? I've just seen him and I want your opinion.'
>
> Lianne: 'I'm sorry I can't help: I'm on my way out and I'm already very late. I'll be able to see him next week when I've got a space. Let me look in my diary.'
>
> Dr M: 'Oh. The problem is I can't start on treatment until I clarify this diagnosis. And he is pretty bad.' [*manipulative bait … plea to the registrar's guilt*]
>
> Lianne: 'I understand that it's frustrating for both of you,' [*fielding the response*] 'I'll be able to see him next week.'
>
> Dr M: 'It won't take long you know.' [*irrelevant logic*]
>
> Lianne: 'Yes, I know, but I need to get going now. I've got a space next Tuesday morning, I'm able to see him then.'

Dr M finally accepts Lianne's refusal. This is a classic situation when you are likely to be diverted by clever, articulate, but irrelevant argument; or when you could lose your self-confidence if affected by the manipulative 'dig' to your self-esteem, provoking guilt.

One of the most effective things about using repetition in this way is that once you have prepared what you are going to say, you can relax and stay with your prepared argument, without panicking that you will need to think on your feet. However manipulative or bullying the other person is, you know exactly what needs to be said. There may be a situation when both parties are being assertive, in which case neither will want to continue for long, but work towards a compromise fairly quickly.

4 Fielding the response

This I consider one of the most fundamental of all assertive skills. In order successfully to 'field' or 'fog' a response, you need to be able to indicate that you have heard what the other person has said, without getting 'hooked' by what they say. Thus you are able to show that you respect the other person's point of view without necessarily sharing it. In order to communicate effectively, you need to listen and indicate that you have heard what is said and acknowledge it, but stick to your guns. This skill is especially useful when handling direct or indirect criticism. The criticism may be direct, for example:

> 'You are never available when I want to see you.'

or implied:

> 'Why can't Mr X have a home visit?'

In the second instance, the request hides anger, frustration and resentment. You could 'read' behind the statement, so that your response could begin:

> 'I understand/accept that it must be very frustrating for you but … I am unable to arrange a home visit …' (offer an alternative)

Note that you need not be drawn into an explanation unless you choose to do so.

In the first instance, when the criticism is more direct, agree with the statement, which disarms your critic. You are acknowledging the probability that there may be some truth in what is said, while remaining your own judge – a powerful position. For example:

> 'Yes, I am often unavailable for you at short notice; however, I am still not able to deal with your request right now.'

Again, you do not need to justify your position.

Fogging, or fielding the response in this way, allows you to receive criticism comfortably without becoming anxious or defensive. It also gives no reward to those manipulating you through unjustified criticism – people who use criticism to diminish your self-esteem rather than in addressing the issue to help you understand yourself better.

When fielding, you need to be emotionally intelligent, and to be aware of all the verbal and non-verbal messages that are being communicated or leaking out. The other person needs to know that you understand their motives and feelings as well as thought. Listen out for the underlying issues, for example:

> 'You seem very angry/frustrated with me.'

> 'I understand this is a difficult/upsetting situation.'

> 'I accept that it must be very irritating.'

Having shown that you are listening sympathetically, you are then able to continue confidently with your statement or answer; you are demonstrating that you are trying to understand the other person's point of view, but you still hold your own:

> 'How come you can only see my child once a week for treatment when he needs it at least twice weekly?'

You read behind the statement and hear the anger and frustration of a concerned parent. Your response could begin:

> 'I accept that it must be very frustrating for you but … hydrotherapy appointments here are booked once weekly.'

Note that you need not be drawn into an explanation unless you chose to.

5 Negotiate

➤ Be prepared to negotiate for what you want.
➤ Assertion does not mean always getting your own way!
➤ Co-operate, bargain as equals, work as a partnership towards achieving something you both want.
➤ Use tact and forethought.
➤ Empathise, co-operate, trade.
➤ Avoid confrontation.
➤ Seek the common ground.
➤ Aim for a win-win situation.

> 'I can see that you are unhappy about that, but I cannot complete the work today. I could finish it by Tuesday, though.'

Or

> 'I understand that you need someone in post full time, but I did plan to only work for six sessions. Perhaps it would help if I spread those sessions over the whole week rather than working for three days on the trot?'

➤ Listen to the other party's point of view before you are able to bargain.
➤ Make certain that you fully understand the other person's position – ask for clarification if necessary.
➤ Prepare yourself well beforehand, harness the facts and figures that help you in supporting your case.
➤ Make certain that you keep to the point: if you feel the conversation is side tracking, bring the discussion back to the central issue: if necessary use the 'broken record' technique.

Effective negotiation should end with both parties coming to terms with a situation they both feel happy about – neither one is compromised – but this does not always happen. Sometimes one party has to bow down. This does not necessarily mean that one of you has 'lost' if you do not get what you want. Reward yourself for making a courageous effort. For more information on negotiating skills, *see* Chapter 8, Negotiation in Section 2.

6 Compromise

Compromise results when both parties have negotiated from an equal position. When moving towards a workable compromise, a solution is found that takes the needs of both parties into consideration.

➤ Do not wait for the other person to give in first: offer a compromise.
➤ Bargain for material goods, but never compromise on your self-respect.
➤ If you feel your personal worth is being questioned, respond as if you are being criticised.
➤ Remain objective and impartial.
➤ You may need to give way to stubbornness; if so, acknowledge this.

There is no compromise about feelings: you have to respect another person's feelings as she or he does your own. Assertive behaviour is fair; there is no win/lose, but a mutually successful outcome. To compromise is to concede, to meet half way. See if you can view compromise as making a virtue of necessity.

7 Accepting criticism

This skill helps you handle constructive criticism from others, by agreeing with or accepting criticism if appropriate instead of reacting to it as if an accusation. Like self-disclosure, this allows you to look more comfortably at the less positive aspects of your own personality or behaviour without denying that that behaviour exists or becoming defensive. At the same time it reduces your critic's hostility. Examples of your response may be:

'Yes, I know I can be aggressive at times.'

'You are right, I am untidy.'

'That's fair enough, I can be indecisive. I'm working on ways to speed up.'

Only agree with the criticism if it is fair or truthful. If you acknowledge the probability of truth in their comment, it disarms the critic, and you demonstrate that you remain your own judge. If someone criticises you directly, learn to acknowledge and agree with the criticism, but only if you feel that the criticism is fair or truthful.

8 Expressing feelings

The importance of understanding and sharing feelings cannot be underestimated in any discussion on assertion.
➤ Learn to identify, or clarify, how we feel before responding to any situation.
➤ Learn to identify what your emotions are telling you.
➤ Talk about your feelings with another person.
➤ Share some of your vulnerability.

Personal exposure does carry a risk; but it is an important part of the openness and honesty of being assertive. There is more about working with feelings in Section 2, Chapter 5.

9   Prompting others to express themselves

This skill allows you more comfortably to seek out criticism about yourself, while prompting the other person to express negative feelings with more honesty. It can improve communication, especially in close relationships, and also encourages your critics to be more assertive. For example, if you suspect that the person you are talking to is hiding her true (negative) feelings, you may ask:

'Are you finding me difficult to talk to?'

'Do you think I am being unfair?'

'Does it seem as though I am pushing you into a corner again?'

'I hear you saying that you think I am disorganised, is that right?'

When behaving assertively, you are confronting issues and situations rather than waiting passively in the hope that you will be able to respond. It is less stressful, and more powerful, to set the agenda yourself.

There are times in any conversation when we suspect that there is something going on beneath the surface. Often it is an intuitive feeling, or a suspicion that something is being said 'between the lines'. At times like this, follow your intuition and take the initiative to seek out, or prompt, an honest response.

10   Listen

➤ The assertive person listens carefully.
➤ Watch and listen to the actual statement, and also for an underlying message.
➤ Learn to 'read' behind the words, and also to watch non-verbal behaviour for 'leakage' or signs that all is not as it seems. For more on non-verbal skills, *see* Section 4.
➤ Clarify or check that you have heard correctly – this is a good way of stalling for time before responding if you cannot identify how you feel about a situation:

'So you think that I ought to be clearer about the facts?'

'Can I just check what you just said? …'

Active listening is a physically demanding, conscious process of attending to what the speaker is saying. It requires the receiver to listen for the total meaning a person conveys – to try to determine both the content of the message and the feelings underlining it. Active listeners note all the cues, both verbal and non-verbal, in communication. When having a conversation with someone, try to spend more time listening than speaking. Let go of those initial urges to speak, and listen more. Listening can take tremendous effort, but each time you train your brain to become slightly more patient.[4]

Good listeners do the following.

➤ Listen: pay close, interested, attention.
➤ Paraphrase: demonstrate they have correctly perceived the sender's inner state and understood: 'Are you saying you dislike that kind of work …?'
➤ Ask questions to clarify the position, or reflect back that you have heard, for example, 'So that made you feel very angry?'
➤ Never interrupt.
➤ Never advise or suggest solutions.
➤ Allow feelings: they do not try not to stop them, but encourage them – suppressing feelings will only increase the sender's discomfort and discourage them from trusting you.

If you feel you may need to improve your listening skills – and most of us do – work with a friend or colleague through the following exercises.

EXERCISE 4

➤ A tells a partner of a true incident that happened to her.
➤ B repeats it, trying to keep the same emphasis and reflection that A had in the telling.
➤ A takes on a different role (e.g. an absent minded older woman) and tells the story again.

Discuss the different impacts within each telling before swapping roles.

EXERCISE 5

One person spends five minutes explaining what she has been doing that day or talking about her last holiday.

The listener demonstrates (by giving verbal and nonverbal cues) that she is listening. After a couple of minutes, she then changes her behaviour to show that she is not listening.

---

4   Alidina S. *Mindfulness for Dummies*. John Wiley & Sons; 2010. pp. 4, 53.

➤ At the end of five minutes the partners swap roles and discuss how it felt to be in each position.
➤ Look at what kinds of behaviour indicate listening/not listening.
➤ What is assertive or aggressive about behaviour in this context?
➤ Discuss how people feel as recipients of each type of behaviour.

EXERCISE 6

Divide into pairs. Spend three minutes each on sharing information either about yourself or a cause you believe in and why.
➤ Summarise what was said.
➤ Listen to each other's summaries.
➤ Discuss any difficulties you had listening to each other and what outside interferences or mannerisms hindered your ability to listen.
➤ Give each other feedback on how they communicated verbally and non-verbally.
➤ Make the feedback constructive and specific, for example, 'It would be better if you talked a little louder', rather than 'You talk too softly' or 'Your voice wasn't right'.

11 Innovate
➤ Take charge and regain control.
➤ Act as your own catalyst for change.
➤ Innovate, and do not wait for others, or fate, to take over.

Some people find that once they are able to let themselves set the scene for change in this way, other areas of their life are affected: they have the confidence to move ahead and perhaps alter the balance of control in their personal as well as professional life. Once you allow yourself to be assertive, you are acknowledging that you are no longer the passive victim of other people's manipulation. You are able to make your own decisions, and this can be a very powerful motivator for change.

12 Empower

Assertiveness is a very powerful and freeing tool. When we behave assertively, we experience very positive feelings, and those feelings inevitably become more meaningful or central to our lives. Assertive behaviour gives us a certain strength and stability; it allows us to have more influence and authority. This extra power is very energetic and potent, but must be used wisely. It is very tempting after years of feeling oppressed or restricted to rush out and regain the world! Allow room for negotiation or compromise.

COMPASSION AND ASSERTION

If you show compassion for the concerns of others, but also communicate your feelings clearly, even strongly, the combination of openheartedness and directness can be very powerful. Compassion and caring support each other: compassion brings caring to assertion, while assertion helps you to feel comfortable giving compassion. Being empathetic can give you lots of useful information about your communication partner – what is really on their mind, what they really care about. In seeing the bigger picture, you reduce any frustration or anger towards them. Empathy does not mean waiving your rights. Any natural capacity for empathy can be strengthened by the following.[5]

➤ Setting the stage – orient yourself to the situation to come.

➤ Stay 'open' and tuned in to the other person.

➤ Notice their actions, the non-verbal communication.

➤ Tune into their expressions and feelings.

➤ Track their thoughts: what might he be feeling here? What could be most important to him? What might he want from me?

➤ Check back: 'Sounds like you are telling me …', 'I get the sense that …'. Or use the format of the positive/negative/positive sandwich. Skill yourself up first so it does not sound formulaic: 'I get that you want X, and that you feel Y about it, but it seemed to me Z, and because I missed getting it right this time, maybe next time chat to me directly about it, because I would love to get this right in future.'

If you find it hard to feel empathy, one of the reasons may be because you are someone who feels their social-emotional capacities are stretched; you may feel overwhelmed when you are with others. If you are mindful of your own emotions, and take care of them, you help heal any shortages of empathy.[6] If this is the case, as you converse, listen well, focus on your own breathing and pay attention to your internal sensations. Use imagery – imagine yourself as a deeply rooted tree or surrounded by a transparent bubble; maybe a picket fence between you and your communication partner, as suggested by Hanson, *et al.*[7]

We have looked at the Personal Bill of Rights in the previous chapter. If you write your own personal code of unilateral, ethical, relationship virtues, you will increase the effectiveness of personal communication.[8] This may look something like:

---

5 Hanson R, Mendius R. *Buddha's Brain: the practical neuroscience of happiness, love and wisdom.* New Harbinger Publications; 2009. pp. 137–8.

6 Siegel DJ. *The Mindful Brain: reflection and attunement in the cultivation of well-being.* WW Norton & Co; 2007. Siegel DJ. *The Developing Mind.* The Guilford Press; 2007.

7 Hanson, Mendius, note 5 above.

8 Ibid. pp. 148–55.

➤ listen, talk less
➤ do not threaten others
➤ say what I need
➤ keep my promises.

In order to communicate compassionately and effectively, you will need to be mindful of, and stay in touch with, deeper feelings and desires. Keep asking yourself what you want/need. You will need to take personal responsibility for getting your needs met in relationships – it will help to take turns to focus on each other's topics when talking, rather than mixing them together. With this in mind, never try to communicate with the aim to fix, change or convince another person – you can only take responsibility for yourself and your own feelings. Once you become familiar with this way of being, you will feel more able to take responsibility for the other person's issues with you, and to identify what there is to correct on your part. If you keep coming back to your own experience – emotions, underlying hopes and wishes – rather than the other person's actions and your opinions about them, and preface conversations with 'I feel …', you will be 'owning' your own feelings and actions.

Stay guided by your own personal, moral code: avoid language that is fault-finding or inflammatory. If you feel triggered by their interaction or lose your way, try using the logical (pre-frontal cortex) to help you – write down the key points in advance. During the conversation, it will help if you focus clearly on the present and future, not the past.

Give yourself time. Remember that whatever is happening is impermanent – consider if you will feel as charged about this in 10 years' time.

Once you have developed a stronger and more empathic communication style, you will find that, over time, truths about other people become apparent. Does this person respect your boundaries? Keep agreements and promises? Repair misunderstandings? If not, consider minimising contact. Hanson says:

> 'A relationship that is bigger than it's real foundation is a set-up for disappointment and hurt, while a relationship that's smaller than it's foundation is a lost opportunity.'[9]

For example, you cannot make a co-worker stop being rude to you, but you can 'shrink' the relationship by minimising your contact with them.

Assertiveness helps you to stick up for yourself and others, and to feel confident that you can still get your needs met even while being compassionate. Be guided by virtue and principle, which regulate more healthy aims. If you stay bound by the key principles of being open to people, non-judgmental, staying

---

9   Hanson, Mendius, note 5 above, p. 152.

connected, alert and awake to possibility, you will be able to communicate more peacefully, with clarity, insight and understanding. When we behave assertively it allows us to have more influence and authority both within our professional role and as human beings. In learning to be assertive, you are releasing untapped potential and beginning a process of self-discovery through which you can begin to understand yourself, and others, more. Through being assertive you also empower others, allowing them the room to take space and negotiate their needs. As your sensitivity to others increases, so will your ability to feel care and compassion.

Use these skills wisely, and recognise that the learning process is slow. Assertiveness is something that takes many, many years to effect – after all, you are learning to undo several years' worth of habitually different behaviour. So go slowly, and accept that in learning to be assertive you are beginning a process of self-discovery through which you can begin to understand your true potential.

KEY POINTS

➤ In learning how to become assertive, habitual ways of communicating will be changed, and this needs courage, determination and practice.

➤ The work is based on testing beliefs and assumptions, and identifying how some of our usually unquestioned thoughts are distorted, unrealistic and unhelpful.

➤ The entirety of our adult life is spent making personal decisions and choices. If we accept this, then we are free and empowered to accept any consequences of our decisions.

➤ We need to protect and take care of ourselves by setting personal boundaries – we need to be able to tell other people when they are acting in ways that are not acceptable to us.

➤ We need to acknowledge and understand our own feelings, to 'own' our own voice and the right to speak up for ourselves.

➤ Assertiveness is a very powerful and freeing tool. When we behave assertively, we experience very positive feelings, and those feelings inevitably become more meaningful, or central to our lives. This extra power is very energetic and potent, but must be used wisely.

➤ Compassion brings caring to assertion, while assertion helps you feel comfortable giving compassion.

➤ In order to communicate compassionately and effectively, you will need to be mindful of, and stay in touch with, deeper feelings and desires. Keep coming back to your own experience rather than the other person's actions, and you will be 'owning' your own feelings and actions.

➤ Stay guided by your own personal moral code.

➤ You will find that, over time, truths about other people become apparent. Does this person respect your boundaries? Keep agreements and promises? Repair misunderstandings? If not, consider minimising contact.

➤ If we stay bound by the key principles of being open to people, non-judgmental, staying connected, alert and awake to possibility, you will be able to communicate more peacefully, with clarity, insight and understanding.

➤ Through being assertive you also empower others, allowing them the room to take space and negotiate their needs.

➤ The assertive speaker is prepared to:
  - be clear and specific
  - be honest and open about your feelings
  - negotiate
  - repeat your message if misunderstood
  - compromise if it is reasonable to do so
  - listen, 'field or fog'
  - self-disclose: express their feelings
  - innovate: take chances and risks
  - accept criticism where appropriate
  - prompt others to express themselves honestly
  - innovate, empower.

FURTHER READING

Back K, Back K. *Assertiveness at Work: a practical guide to handling awkward situations.* 3rd ed. McGraw-Hill Professional; 2005.

Bishop S. *Develop Your Assertiveness.* 2nd ed. Kogan Page; 2006.

Hadfield S, Hasson G. *How to be Assertive in Any Situation.* Pearson Life; 2012.

Lindenfield G. *Assert Yourself: a self help assertiveness programme for men and women.* Thorsons; 1992.

Potts S. *Entitled to Respect: how to be confident and assertive in the workplace.* How To Books Ltd; 2010.

Smith MJ. *When I Say No I Feel Guilty.* Bantam USA; 1975.

CHAPTER 4

Putting your ideas into practice

In this chapter we look at the sets of skills needed to make the changes required to become more assertive. We are all very different, with different skills and abilities, and we achieve at different rates. Research on success in reaching goals suggests that self-efficacy best explains why people with the same level of knowledge and skills get very different results. According to researchers,[1] self-confidence functions as a powerful predictor of success because it makes you expect to succeed: it allows you take risks and set challenging goals, it helps you keep trying if at first you do not succeed, and it helps you control emotions and fears when the going gets rough.

How likely are we to achieve? There seems to be a set of human strengths that are the most likely buffers against mental illness: courage, optimism, interpersonal skill, work ethic, hope, honesty and perseverance.[2] It may be that these skills are the ones needed to be fostered in order to be able to work on developing a new set of skills such as those needed to be assertive. It is also helpful to challenge yourself with encouragement and positivity: too many of us tell ourselves 'I am going to do this and do it right', 'I should focus 100%', 'I am going to try extra hard'. A better attitude may be to foster thoughts from the Mindfulness literature:[3] ' I will treat myself kindly, and acknowledge whatever my experience is, I will try as best I can/I won't try too hard, nor give up, I'll stay somewhere in the middle.' It is worth remembering that sometimes when we stop trying to change things, they change by themselves.

That said, any sort of development, organisational or personal, requires a framework if we wish to know whether change has actually occurred. In the case of personal development, we often function as the primary judge of our own improvement, but validation of objective improvement requires assessment using standard criteria. Personal development frameworks ideally need to include goals or benchmarks that define the end-points; strategies and plans for reaching goals; measurement and assessment of progress, levels or stages that define milestones along a development path; and a feedback system to provide information on changes.

---

1 Bandura A. *Self-Efficacy: the exercise of control*. WH Freeman and Co.; 1988. p. 184.
2 Seligman MEP. Building human strength: psychology's forgotten mission. *APA Monitor*. **29**(1).
3 Alidina S. *Mindfulness for Dummies*. John Wiley & Sons; 2010. pp. 1, 16.

SETTING GOALS

If you want to change the way you behave, or change the way you think about things, your goals need to be SMART, focussed. Use principles based on the SMART technique[4] to help you define these goals. There is no clear consensus about what the SMART acronym means, or even what it is in any given situation. Wade and others have summarised the words associated with the SMART acronym that appear in the literature.[5] The lack of consensus highlights the intrinsic difficulty in using this particular framework as a clinical standard, but for our purpose here, typically accepted values are:

S	Specific	Significant, Stretching, Simple
M	Measurable	Meaningful, Motivational, Manageable
A	Attainable	Appropriate, Achievable, Agreed, Assignable, Actionable, Ambitious, Aligned, Aspirational, Acceptable, Action-focused
R	Relevant	Results-oriented, Resourced, Resonant, Realistic
T	Timely	Time-oriented, Time framed, Timed, Time-based, Time-boxed, Time-bound, Time-specific, Timetabled, Time limited, Trackable, Tangible
E	Evaluate	Ethical, Excitable, Enjoyable, Engaging, Ecological
R	Re-evaluate	Rewarded, Reassess, Revisit, Recordable, Rewarding, Reaching

Try to set your goals using words that are meaningful to you, or, if working with a client, the client.

S   Be *Specific* – the goals must be clear and concrete: 'I will practise saying "no".'

M   Make sure they are *Measurable* – identify markers that will indicate when you have reached your goals: 'I will keep a notebook noting daily successes.'

A   *Achievable* – ensure that your goals are realistic. Ask yourself the question of whether your goal is actually achievable or not, and be honest! 'I will practise saying "no" to unachievable demands set on me at work, to family and baby sitting, but need to think more about how to manage it with my mother …'

---

4   Doran GT. There's a SMART way to write management's goals and objectives. *Management Review.* 1981; **70**(11) [AMA forum]: 35–6.
5   Wade D. Goal setting in rehabilitation: an overview of what, why and how [editorial]. *Clinical Rehabilitation.* 2009; **23**(4): 291–5.

R *Relevant/realistic* – choose goals that are applicable to your personal development. Make sure that these goals are something you are truly invested in, because you will be focusing a great deal of time and energy on them.

T *Time-related* – set a timeline that will guide your progress. Specifying a goal for two years down the road is not as powerful a motivator as one that you set for the next six months.

The goal you set must be challenging. At the same time, it should be realistic and attainable, not impossible to reach. It should be challenging enough to make you stretch, but not so far that you break.[6]

You need to think about what you want to achieve over the long and short term, and to be specific about the losses and gains. You need to look clearly at the outcome you want to achieve, and also to be clear about what you want to do toward achieving your goal on a daily basis. Learning to change your behaviour is hard work! But you can get there, with focus and determination. Here are a few suggested routes.

1   Goal setting

Goals give us something to work toward, and help us to feel that we are moving along a specific path. Establishing goals invites us to look at the big picture, break it down into smaller pieces and get started toward accomplishing our important hopes and dreams. There is often uncertainty about how to set goals. One of the most common problems is that the goals tend to be too big. It is much easier to achieve smaller goals that fit with a larger objective than to try to accomplish everything all at once. The following process may help you formulate your plans.

2   Lifetime goals

When thinking about what you want to achieve over the long and short term, break your thinking down a little more to be specific about the losses and gain. Look clearly at the outcome you want to achieve, and also be clear about what you want to do toward achieving your goal on a daily basis. Here is one suggested model, taken from the neuro-linguistic programming literature.[7]

Where are you now?

Take charge of your life and look at all the areas of your life, considering those you feel you want to change. How happy are you with these areas of your life? Give yourself a score out of 10. Here are some suggested areas to begin with.

6   Hanson R, Mendius R. *Buddha's Brain: the practical neuroscience of happiness, love and wisdom.* New Harbinger Publications; 2009.

7   Ready R, Burton K. In: Miller W, Rollnick S, editors. *Neurolinguistic Programming for Dummies: taking charge of your life.* The Guilford Press; 2002. Ch. 3, pp. 36–45.

Home environment/house/garden 1...2...3...4...5...6...7...8...9...10	**Charitable giving/voluntary work/kindness/giving of self to others** 1...2...3...4...5...6...7...8...9...10
Finances and money 1...2...3...4...5...6...7...8...9...10	**Friendships** 1...2...3...4...5...6...7...8...9...10
Spirituality/religion 1...2...3...4...5...6...7...8...9...10	**Relationship/sex/loving** 1...2...3...4...5...6...7...8...9...10
Health/exercise/weight 1...2...3...4...5...6...7...8...9...10	**Family** 1...2...3...4...5...6...7...8...9...10
Fun, home, recreation, leisure time 1...2...3...4...5...6...7...8...9...10	**Creativity** 1...2...3...4...5...6...7...8...9...10
Work/career 1...2...3...4...5...6...7...8...9...10	**Therapy/personal growth** 1...2...3...4...5...6...7...8...9...10

Having noted where you are now, note what you want to achieve over a *lifetime*. What number do you think is attainable? What about 10 years? Five years? Now consider your *short term goals* – more tangible, six months to one year perhaps.

Setting the goals
➤ Make them SMART.
➤ Make sure they are self-initiated, maintained and within your control.
➤ State them positively: 'I will, I can …'
➤ Check whether the goals are within your control to effect.
➤ Describe the content: 'Who/why/what/where/when can this be achieved? What will I want to do with it?'
➤ Does a goal identify any required resources? People, money, time?
➤ Does it identify the first step you need to take?
➤ How will you know the outcome? 'How will I see it, smell it, hear or feel it?'
➤ Will there be any secondary gains? 'How will this benefit the environment, my family, friends? Will I save money? Who else will be happy?'
➤ Make a list of the losses and gains if you achieve the goal.
➤ What would happen if you achieve your goal, and if you do not? Make that list.

Reward yourself
➤ Keep a diary of your progress and revisit it monthly.
➤ Tell your friends.
➤ Focus on the benefits of success.

3 Challenging negative beliefs

If you are nervous about trying out some of the ideas in this book, you may need a practise run. You could either role play with some colleagues or friends, or try a dummy run and note what happens. If you have a tendency towards passivity and are avoiding trying out some of the assertiveness techniques, try some of the following ideas, which are strategies developed from psychological practice, primarily cognitive behaviour therapy (CBT).

CBT is based on the theory that much of our anxious and worry behaviour is a result of problematic thoughts (cognitions) and behaviours, and that if these are targeted such thoughts can be overcome. It uses commonsense ideas to allow you to experiment safely and test what works and what does not, and whether your predictions of failure actually materialise or, more likely, you achieve and move on. Use these methods to find out what works and what does not work for you. You can also use the principles to manage change in clients and patients you are working with. This formula takes principles from CBT individual and group treatment programmes.[8]

Your experimental record book for challenging negative beliefs

There are three main principles to follow here:
➤ notice and note you have a belief
➤ you challenge this belief
➤ you experiment with the belief.

There is a particular method to this. Pick a situation that you worry you would not be able to deal with in the past or present. Say you are a newly qualified practitioner and feel ready to work without supervision now, after only four months. You have a belief that you could never tell your supervisor that you feel ready to be signed off – you worry that they would challenge you or think you arrogant. You that worry they might tell you all the reasons why you are not ready yet.

How much you believe this – 10%? 50%? 85%?

Now challenge or dispute this belief. Take it apart. How accurate is it? Get to the facts.

Challenging the belief

Examine the evidence for and against.

Evidence for
➤ What makes you think you could never do this?
➤ How does not doing this help you cope or solve the problem?

---

8 Nathan P, Smith L, Rees C, *et al*. *Mood management Course: a cognitive behavioural group treatment programme for anxiety and depression*. 2nd ed. Centre for Clinical Interventions; 2004.

➤ Where is the evidence for this belief?
➤ Is it good, solid and reliable evidence?
➤ Is there any other way you could view this evidence for yourself?

Evidence against
➤ Have there been times when you have been told you are not ready for something and you felt foolish or overly criticised?
➤ What are the disadvantages of not acting?
➤ Have there been situations when you have acted, and it all turned out ok?
➤ What happened? Did you get a compliment for your work so far? Was your teacher/supervisor disgusted with you? Were you uncontrollably angry/upset? Did you stumble/cry/break down/lose control? What are the facts?

Example

Evidence for	Evidence against
The fact that nothing bad ever happens is because I do not act on anything.	I actually get into trouble for not showing/demonstrating a level of competence, and am seen perhaps to rely too much on waiting to be told what to do. I may justly be criticised for not being proactive enough, for not following things through confidently and competently, even though I know I can do it.
What actually happened?	
Before I spoke with my supervisor, I felt awful – it was easier to let it go, even though the feelings kept resurfacing. I imagined she would laugh at me, or report me, and maybe even extend my probationary period. She would definitely not like me for challenging her judgement.	When I did speak to her, it was fine. I felt uncomfortable to begin with, but it was good seeing her understand that I was ready: I had prepared some strategies to try and we worked out a plan of action should I feel I need some help. She felt confident I was ready, as I had shown her I was happy to take up the challenge.

Experiment with your belief

Set some time aside to focus on your beliefs, challenge them, looking at the evidence.

Rate again how much you believe that the situation you worry about you would not be able to deal with. Could you now take more charge of your needs/feel confident to assert them in the future? Could you practise another specific assertiveness skill in real life?

How much you believe this – 10%? 50%? 85%?

If there is a weakening, however small, of your central belief, congratulate yourself. If there is no change yet, do not panic! Changing your beliefs takes time and persistence. Keep practising the strategy. A good gauge of when you have done enough work is when your belief is relatively weak, perhaps 20%.

If you keep a record of your experiences, or experiments, you will be able to test your hypothesis and see if your predictions were true. These behaviour experiments may also show you that your negative expectations and predictions do not actually come true. Unfortunately, we are hard-wired to believe more in our negative than positive predictions about the world, as a throw-back to the times when fearful alertness to our environment could be life-saving. Potential threats were round every corner, and our brains have evolved to be hyper-vigilant and automatically predict this. Our brains typically detect negative information faster than positive,[9] so it is important to reverse any negative predictions and demonstrate to ourselves what has worked – as otherwise we will slip back into our usual negative belief structures.

Research has shown also that appraising a situation more accurately leads to more positive emotions and fewer negative ones.[10] Not only will doing something and moving forward make you feel better, it will almost always improve a situation that is worrying you.[11] So on every level it makes sense to record your practice in this way.

Here is another way you could record your work.

1	Prediction	I could never ask X to cover my shift again. (85% impossible)
2	Experiment	In the staff room, during day shift (make sure we are alone), I will apologise for messing X about last time and ask.
3	Record	I felt sick before, couldn't get X alone, but I did it, and she was fine: we negotiated some mutually useful swaps over the next month.
4	Conclusion	I can do it! My theory was X would be angry and I would lose my friendship. New conviction: 95% in favour of asking
5	Next steps	Try in more difficult circumstance: ask M if I can reduce my hours permanently. Offer some solutions/benefits to her in the negotiation.

9 Yang E, Zald DH, Blake R. Fearful expressions gain preferential access to awareness during continuous flash suppression. *Emotion*. 2007; **7**(4): 882–6.

10 Gross JJ, John OP. Individual differences in two emotion regulation processes: implications for affect, relationships, and well-being. *Journal of Personality and Social Psychology*. 2003; **85**: 348–62.

11 Aspinwall LG, Taylor SE. A stitch in time: self-regulation and proactive coping. *Psychological Bulletin*. 1997; **121**: 417–36.

1   Prediction

Here, you need to begin by being clear and specific about the negative or different predictions you are testing. Outline the thought or belief you are testing and rate your strength of conviction between 0 and 100%.

2   Experiment

Decide and plan what you will do. Be very specific and include *what* you will do, *who* you will do it with, *where*, *when* and *how*. Consider whether you may meet any obstacles, and how you will overcome them. Plan what you will do if your prediction comes true, for example, how will you respond assertively if someone is critical of you? How will you measure your results?

3   Record your results

Make a note of what actually happened, using clear, observable outcomes. Include your thoughts, feelings, any physical sensations and what the other people did. As you verbally describe what you are feeling to yourself, you increase frontal lobe regulation of the limbic system, enabling you to feel calmer and in control.[12]

4   Conclusion

Use this column to record your conclusion and write any comments. Evaluate the results. Check you are not being biased! What have you learned about your predictions? Where they accurate? Has your theory changed in the light of the results? Re-rate your original strength of conviction in percentage terms.

5   The future

Plan ways you can consolidate what you have discovered. For example, should you repeat it, or try another one? Do it differently? Try to stretch yourself, try a new way.

Example

Rosa was a well-respected and well-liked physiotherapist working in an acute rehabilitation unit, but she often avoided standing up for herself and her beliefs when challenged, as she hated conflict and felt unequal to managing it. Consequently, she would always take the easy way out of difficult situations. Fundamentally, she wanted to be liked. Her biggest complaint, second to the fact that she never seemed to get promoted, was that people described her as 'too nice'. She had been working on developing assertiveness skills for a while, and here she set

---

12 Lieberman MD, Eisenberger NI, Crockett MJ, *et al.* Putting feelings into words. Affect labeling disrupts amygdala activity in response to affective stimuli. *Association for Psychological Science.* 2007; **18**(5): 421–8.

herself the challenge of discharging a child (P) with cerebral palsy whose mother led the local action group for children with disabilities. In the previous session, when Rosa had mooted the idea of a future discharge, the mother said she 'disagreed' and would 'fight tooth and nail' against any discharge. Rosa discussed this in supervision, and decided that she would take up the challenge and continue with her plans to discharge P. Here is her thinking afterwards.

Evidence for not doing anything – keeping the status quo	Evidence against
The fact that nothing bad ever happens is because I do not act on anything.	I actually get into trouble for not discharging enough patients, and not being proactive enough, for not following things through.
Before I discharged P I felt awful, I felt I was going to let Mum down and felt sure there were other things we could offer her if only I knew about them.	When I did discharge P, it was fine. I felt uncomfortable to begin with, but it was good seeing Mum understand that she had some strategies to try and she felt more in control of how to help P.

Rosa's comments/learning points
➤ I couldn't have done this without supervision.
➤ I could have done with a bit of role play, but I used the 'stuck record' technique effectively when Mum tried to side-track me.
➤ I took a list of strategies that Mum could follow with me. Without those I might not have been able to continue with confidence.

Next steps
➤ I will aim to discharge five more of my long-standing patients/clients with the next month.
➤ I will use the same technique until I feel totally comfortable, then I may try another one.
➤ I will try this technique with a slightly more difficult situation within the next three months.

There are many other ways to work with challenging our central, core beliefs, and for those of you wanting to explore this I recommend the excellent *Therapy for Dummies* series.[13] CBT therapists encourage you to challenge core beliefs, and eventually this process can become second nature as the concepts become incorporated into your new ways of thinking: after all, it is reflective thinking.

13 Willson R, Branch R. *Cognitive Behaviour Therapy for Dummies*. John Wiley & Sons; 2006. Alidina S. *Mindfulness for Dummies*. John Wiley & Sons; 2010. Ready R, Burton K. *Neurolingusitic Programming for Dummies*. John Wiley & Sons; 2010.

KEY POINTS

➤ We are all very different, with different skills and abilities, and achieve at different rates.

➤ Expect to succeed: it allows you take risks and set challenging goals; it helps you keep trying; and it helps you control emotions and fears when the going gets rough.

➤ Buffer yourself with courage, optimism, interpersonal skill, work ethic, hope, honesty and perseverance. Treat yourself kindly.

➤ Any sort of development requires a framework so we know whether change has actually occurred. Include goals or benchmarks that define the end-points; strategies and plans for reaching goals; measurement and assessment of progress, levels or stages that define milestones along a development path; and a feedback system to provide information on changes.

➤ Use principles based on the SMART technique to help you define these goals: Specific, measurable, achievable, realistic, timed. State them positively, Describe the content and if it needs any resources. How will you know the outcome? Make a list of the losses and gains if you achieve your goal, and reward yourself.

➤ Challenge negative beliefs. Notice you have a belief, challenge this, and experiment with it. Look for the evidence for and against the belief. Rate how much you believe it. Our brains typically detect negative information faster than positive, so it is important to reverse any negative predictions and demonstrate to ourselves what has worked – as otherwise we will slip back into our usual negative belief structures.

➤ Appraising a situation more accurately leads to more positive emotions and fewer negative ones. Doing something and moving forward will almost always improve a situation that is worrying you.

➤ Record your work:

☐ *Prediction*	☐ *Experiment*	☐ *Record*	☐ *Conclude*	☐ *Next steps*

➤ Reflect. Write down, use tables, columns or mind mapping, whichever suits your own learning style. Soon you will be able to reflect without resorting to pen and paper. Challenge the doubts. Identify what gets in the way of you achieving your aim. Examine your commitment to change, and identify when, where, how and who can help you work on it. Keep a diary or success chart to help keep you motivated.

FURTHER READING

Beck AT. *Cognitive Therapy and the Emotional Disorders*. Penguin Psychology; 1991.
Beck JS. *Cognitive Therapy: basics and beyond*. The Guilford Press; 1995.

Ellis A. *Reason and Emotion in Psychotherapy: a comprehensive method for treating human disturbances*. Revised and updated. Birch Lane Press; 1995.

Willson R, Branch R. *Cognitive Behaviour Therapy for Dummies*. John Wiley & Sons; 2006.

Ready R, Burton K. *Neurolingusitic Programming for Dummies*. John Wiley & Sons; 2010.

Section 2

Assertiveness in practice

CHAPTER 5

Feelings

We begin this section by referring back to Chapters 3 and 4, remembering that, in working with behavioural change such as learning assertiveness skills, we need to address the way we think and behave in response to situations and to develop more flexible ways to think and reason. However, if we just work on behavioural output there is a possibility the change will be artificial, and superficial. For real change to occur we need to incorporate some personal awareness work, and make our unconscious more conscious: we need the conscious work to gain insight into our unconscious emotions and drives.

Part of this work will be to notice and overcome our personal difficulties by identifying and changing dysfunctional thinking, behaviour and emotional responses. We will need to gain awareness of, and test our beliefs and assumptions about, ourselves. We need to gain awareness and understanding of our feelings, how we operate and are seen by others, and identify how some of our usually unquestioned thoughts, behaviours and immediate responses – which are possibly dysfunctional, unrealistic or unhelpful. Once those thoughts have been acknowledged and challenged, our feelings and behaviours have a chance to change fundamentally, not just superficially.

In this chapter we look at the importance of identifying feelings clearly before responding to a situation. We need to look at why this skill is so important and why it is something that many of us find so difficult.

In order to understand ourselves fully, we need to be prepared to explore our darker side. We also need to work at understanding how others are different from us. Other people have different tastes, personalities, values and judgements. This ability to have empathy for difference, to be open to diversity, to work hard at noticing difference, is crucial to the work of being assertive. It will help you to look at the way you interpret things, how you plan and engage in behaviour that is likely to be useful to you, and help you to develop your skills and abilities.

It is crucial too to look at our feelings, and ourselves, with compassion and mindful acceptance, to accept our painful thoughts and feelings rather than over-identifying with them: our feeling and experiences are part of the human condition, not personal, isolating or shameful. We need to understand our own difficulties and be kind and warm to ourselves in the face of failure and setbacks rather than be harshly judgmental and self-critical. Learning more about how to accept ourselves and others with compassion[1] may help here.

If we learn to develop self-compassion, and direct our attention and focus on the positive within ourselves rather than the negative, we have a better chance of positive changes in our behaviour and our relationship with ourselves. To do this, we need to think and reason (about others, ourselves, and our relationships) and behave in ways that we identify will be helpful. This can range from simply being kind to ourselves – building in adequate 'time out', a bath, a day of self-indulgence or a holiday – or it may require courage to do things that are blocking us from developing. In thinking about some of your patterns of behaviour, try to develop a sensory focus: feel and use imagery with warmth, support and kindness. Do not give yourself a hard time!

If we are vulnerable to shame, or tend towards perfection, we may attack ourselves ('I should have done better', 'What's the matter with me?'), attack others ('Why is it me that always has to remember everything?'), or simply give up ('There's nothing I can do, there's no point in trying'). None of these are useful. Paradoxically, here the key to success is the ability to engage your cognition and intellect and rely less on feeling and more on rational thought. For example, if you are feeling disappointed, it is good to acknowledge that, but then move on and deal with the disappointment more practically, instead of staying with the disappointment, noting 'this situation threatens me because …'[2]

It is important to verbalise feelings, and to precede statements with 'I feel'. When we say 'I am angry, I'm hurt', etc., we are stating that the feeling is who we are. But emotions do not define us; they are a form of internal communication that helps us to understand ourselves. They are a vital part of our being – as a component of the whole. This is 'owning' the feeling. By stating the feeling we affirm that we have a right to feelings. We are affirming it to ourselves – and taking responsibility for owning ourselves and our reality. It is important that our communication partners can hear and understand us, but it is not as important as hearing ourselves and understanding that we have a right to our feelings. It is vitally important to own our own voice, to 'own' our right to speak up for ourselves.

EMOTIONS AND FEELINGS

To begin some of this work, notice how emotions tie up with a physical feeling. Research has shown us that our guts contain cerebral neurological tissue – a mass the size of a cat's brain. Hence the term – 'a gut feeling'. To help us identify how we feel, it is useful to honour and acknowledge this, and use all our senses

---

1 Gilbert P. *The Compassionate Mind*. Kindle ed. Constable; 2010. pp. 71, 219.
2 Ibid. p. 362.

to help define how we feel through the innate use of intuition. If we connect with our senses – sight, sound, touch, smell and taste – we will make a sensible decision ('I sense something's wrong', 'She's come to her senses'). We need to pay attention to information/stimulation coming from our senses as well as our thoughts and emotions.[3]

Think of when you feel you are understood, and have recognisable choice. Conversely, how do you feel when you are not loved or understood? Try to identify the physical feeling that goes with the emotion.

EXERCISE 1

How do you feel when?

Feeling	Emotions	Physical	Without	Feeling
Loved	Happy/confident	Warm/energetic	Insecure/rejected	Sick and tense when unloved
Understood				
Given choice				

EXERCISE 2

List all the positive and negative things you can think of about each of these people in turn.

Mother

Positive	Negative	Feeling?
Good sense humour	Can be insensitive to my feelings	

Father

Positive	Negative	Feeling?
Generous	Very stubborn	

---

3   Alidina S. *Mindfulness for Dummies*. John Wiley & Sons; 2010. para. 2.25.

Sibling

Positive	Negative	Feeling?

Friend

Positive	Negative	Feeling?

Mr/Ms Difficult at work

Positive	Negative	Feeling?
Thoughtful about patients	Thoughtless around staff	

Mr/Ms Easy

Positive	Negative	Feeling?

Are there any links? Here you are beginning to look to your roots and ingrained, habitual feelings. Are there any similarities between people? What pushes your buttons the most?

Transactional analysis

Some of our feelings are generated by the re-stimulation of old 'scripts', old and familiar ways of being in the world. It makes sense that some of our adult patterns of life or behaviour originated in childhood. We often continue to replay childhood strategies, even when this results in pain or defeat. Eric Berne's research led him to this conclusion, and to theorise that we all have three 'ego states' – parent, child, adult – and that it is these three states that determine how we act, interact and react to others.[4] The model helps to explain how people function and express their personality in their behaviour.

---

4   Berne E. *Transactional Analysis in Psychotherapy: a systematic individual and social psychiatry.* Grove Press; 1961. pp. 232–46. Berne E. *Games People Play: the psychology of human relationships.* Penguin; 2010.

Transactional analysis (TA) is an integrative psychological approach which uses elements of psychoanalytic, humanist and cognitive approaches. According to the International Transactional Analysis Association, TA is 'a theory of personality and a systematic psychotherapy for personal growth and personal change'.[5] It is also a theory of communication, and one that we will return to in other sections of the book. In practice, it provides a method of therapy for individuals, couples, families and groups.

At any given time, a person experiences and manifests their personality through a mixture of behaviours, thoughts and feelings. Typically, according to TA, there are three ego states that people consistently use.

➤ **Parent:** a state in which people behave, feel and think in response to an unconscious mimicking of how their parents (or other parental figures) acted, or how they interpreted their parent's actions.

➤ **Adult:** a state of the ego which is most like a computer processing information and making predictions ; without the major emotions that could affect its operation. Learning to strengthen the adult is a goal of TA. While a person is in the adult ego state, he or she is directed towards an objective appraisal of reality.

➤ **Child:** a state in which people behave, feel and think similarly to how they did in childhood. For example, a person who is criticised at work may respond by looking at the floor and pouting, as they used to when scolded as a child. Conversely, a person who receives a good evaluation may respond with a broad smile and a joyful gesture of thanks. The child is the source of emotions, creation, recreation, spontaneity and intimacy.

The theory states that when in 'parent' we can feel and behave in either nurturing (caring and supportive) or critical (condescending and judgmental) ways; as 'child' in either adapted (compliant, defiant or complaining) or free (curious, fun loving, spontaneous) ways. Berne feels we need to find the 'adult' in ourselves, and behave instead in an open-minded, but logical, interested way to events and life around us.

If we feel *critical*, or we notice others are behaving critically, we are likely to see this both verbally and non-verbally through judgmental behaviour – finger pointing, furrowed brow, with words such as 'ought, must, should'. Conversely, the ego state of *nurturing parent* leads us to relaxed, smiley, attentive behaviour. In our *adult* state, we are more conscious, analytical, centred, relaxed and attentive, and thus use logical terminology like 'who/why/what/where/when' to establish facts.

---

5 Stewart I, Joines V. *TA Today: a new introduction to transactional analysis.* 2nd revised ed. Lifespace Publishing; 2012.

The TA hypothesis is that if we encounter someone whose behaviour reminds us of a critical, or nurturing, parent, we automatically adapt by reacting, behaving in an old familiar way – our childish way – by interacting in either adapted or free child. Conversely, if we behave in either an authoritarian or nurturing way, our communication partner will rise to the bait and respond emotionally accordingly – depending on their dominant ego state. These responses are termed 'transactions', and we will refer to this later in the chapter. For our purposes, we focus here on gaining awareness, and beginning to identify the source of our feelings and responses.

EXERCISE 3

Noting and naming the feelings

➤ List five things that make you feel angry, for example, 'people who swear'.
➤ List five things that make you feel hurt, for example, 'people who ignore me'.
➤ List five things that make you feel happy, for example, 'people who respect my need for privacy'.
➤ List five things that make you feel irritated, for example, 'people who push in a queue'.

EXERCISE 4

1. Use a mind map and write down the trigger at the top that makes you feel anxious or upset (talking to my manager, giving a presentation, phoning my dad).
2. In the central circle, write down any key thoughts or meanings you attach to the trigger (I am going to get angry, fail, become speechless, etc.).
3. Continue using a mind-mapping technique, and write down your emotions (e.g. guilt, fear, panic) any physical sensations (sickness, palpitations, stomach ache).
4. Write down any useful and not so useful behaviours (slamming the phone down, taking a sip of water or deep breath.
5. Think about what you are focusing your attention on most, and consider if this is a useful thing or not (focus on how dizzy I feel versus focus on my quiet breathing).

EXERCISE 5

Think of three or four recent difficult encounters you have had with other people.

Situation	My verbal response	My body language	My feelings	What I really wanted to say/do	How I would have chosen to handle the situation assertively

To behave assertively, we need to verbalise, act on and hence release feelings. This is difficult for all of us in Western culture because, to some extent, free expression of feeling in adulthood is discouraged, and intellectual and rational 'adult' behaviour predominate and are valued. Emotion or intuition still tend to be seen as 'female' and hence devalued in favour of the more 'male' states: adults are supposed to be in control, so negative feelings are often suppressed to the detriment of our emotional and physical health.

Assertiveness experts, including Dickson,[6] note that feelings are physiological events that happen inside our bodies, but 'we talk of becoming "overpowered" by rage or "beside ourselves" with anger, which reinforces the idea that these feelings are somehow detached from us'. However, given that feelings actually generate changes in our body chemistry, if we listen to our 'gut feelings', symptoms such as a lump in the throat, a pounding heart, sinking stomach or sweaty palms, we know that our body is communicating effectively, and we can build on that.

SOME FACTS ABOUT FEELINGS

Dickson and others have noted some facts about feelings.[7]

Personal responsibility

We cannot be held responsible for our feelings, as we cannot stop our body reacting; but we can take charge of how we act on those feelings by verbalising and sharing feeling, telling others when we feel sad, angry, envious or unsure. Although people can argue with your logic, they cannot deny or dismiss your feelings. You have a right to them.

---

6   Dickson A, Charlesworth K. *A Woman in Your Own Right: assertiveness and you*. Quartet Books; 1982.
7   Ibid.

Releasing stress

It is thought that feelings not released can accumulate, leading to accumulated stress. Certainly, any work on noting and allowing feelings can be cathartic, freeing. There is some debate about the usefulness of releasing feelings physically, but there is no harm in naming the feeling appropriately. If you are provoked to anger during a meeting, it may be appropriate simply to state your truth. Feelings can be diffused: if you understand and acknowledge them, it helps to release and dissipate the chemical build up. By verbalising feelings, one takes a risk and shares something very personal, and there is a high chance that others will be freed up to do the same. This personal exposure enhances and builds relationships.

The irrationality of feelings

Feelings often conflict with what we think is rational. If your present reaction seems inappropriate, you could be responding to something unresolved from your past. It may help to understand what is behind the feeling: sadness, or loss? If, for example, your parents were over-critical when you were young, it may be especially difficult for you to accept criticism from authority figures now. Here you need to identify and not dismiss the feeling in the hope it will go away. Correct identification of a feeling such as humiliation or anger can lead to its resolution.

Feelings and choice

We need to be able to make choices in our lives. If this need is blocked, we experience frustration, helplessness, irritation, anger. If the need if fulfilled, we feel powerful, enthused and energised. One of the reasons why morale is so low in the public sector at present is because that need to make choices and change things is being cramped by government dictates. There is frustration with a lack of funding and time, and with unsympathetic or badly informed management. We are all familiar with the feelings of helplessness and outrage that result.

We need to feel understood

If this need is satisfied, we feel secure, safe and valued. If not, feelings range from feeling isolated and fearful to anxious, panicky and confused. If we feel our role is misunderstood at work, we seek support and understanding from colleagues in the same profession or position. The depth and quality of that feeling varies depending on how much we identify with our work.

Humans are social beings: we all have a need to give and receive love and friendship

Once this need is fulfilled, we experience closeness, belonging, affection. If denied us, the negative feelings are sadness, rejection, loneliness. Many of us get a great deal of satisfaction from working as a member of a close-knit team. If the team is not cohesive, or you work much of the day in isolation, disharmony of feeling can result.

MANAGING EMOTIONS

The early pioneers of cognitive behaviour therapy discussed how feelings can be expressed at three different levels:
➤ acknowledgement
➤ verbal expression
➤ physical release.

At the *first level*, privately notice and acknowledge what you feel, without verbalising it. Many people experience a time lapse between the experience of an emotional response and the acknowledgement of it. Often the realisation comes later, with a flash of recognition: 'If only I'd said such and such!' With time and practice you will become more adapt at recognising what is going on, and learn to act on it quickly.

At the *second level*, you make a simple statement about how you feel.

> 'I feel very happy/envious.'

> 'That makes me feel very angry.'

> 'I feel hurt by that comment.'

The immediate effect of this is to reduce your anxiety, allowing you to relax and take control.

At the *third level*, feelings are released physically. Find your own way of releasing anger: yelling in the car on the way home, punching a cushion, any way that you find easy to release the adrenaline and frustration. Crying can be a very therapeutic way to release pent-up disappointment or sadness: allow yourself to mourn. Use the information you body is giving you to release the emotions in a safe place.

Feelings are powerful, and negative feelings especially provoke fear. Because we fear their intensity, we often try to harness them, to control them, in order somehow to diminish their power. But once you allow yourself to feel them, they lose their power. Ride with it. Once you have experienced the feeling fully it no longer controls you, it becomes something familiar and therefore less scary. If you cut yourself off from what you feel, not only is this psychologically dangerous, but also you are denying yourself access to your wise inner self, and closing the door to self-expression and fulfilment. The Mindfulness literature[8]

---

8   *See* Alidina, note 3 above.

particularly values noticing, staying with and verbalising feelings ('I feel panicked, scared, anxious'), rather than avoiding them.

Anger

Anger can be positive, powerful and energising, but we are often uncomfortable freely expressing our anger: it can be frightening, and is often equated with aggression, arrogance and un-femininity. However, anger can be a very motivating force: it can motivate us to change things; it gives us the impetus to move direction in life or take up challenges; it can be vigorous, creative and determined. Directed anger can politicise. It makes politicians, charity leaders and many of society's leading figures: it makes doctors, nurses, therapists. Where we feel angry, we express the fact that we care, passionately.

Where anger is devalued it gets suppressed, and it remains for many people one of the most difficult emotions to handle. For many women, it is especially difficult to reveal that side of their nature. Middle- and owning-class women in particular have been socialised and encouraged from childhood to repress 'difficult' (especially noisy) emotions: to be 'ladylike', compassionate and caring. Often it is the women's experience to be told that such behaviour is threatening or domineering; men often equate our anger with hysteria. Because we have not been allowed to experience anger, we fear its effects, and imagine that being angry is like unleashing a wild dog that will provoke violence and destroy everything in its path.

Thus we employ a variety of ways through which we express anger indirectly. We may flare under the slightest provocation, showing that hurt and frustration has been slowly accumulating beneath the surface. We control ourselves and anger eventually emerges as sarcasm or bullying; we bury it, whine or moan. If this happens, we feel irritable, frustrated, tense, spiteful or resentful, impotent, constrained, or aggrieved. When we block our anger, it emerges as aggression, which is a form of badly stifled anger. If we repress it still further, we may respond passively or not at all; this non-response blocks the energy, and the power moves within, holding us back. This form of control is thought to lead us to build up hurts, and the resulting helplessness leads quickly to apathy, resignation and depression. If we understand and express anger assertively, we act to revoke those feelings of resentment and powerlessness and create change in our lives. Once we allow ourselves to express anger, we recall some of that energy, and regain a sense of our own power and purpose.

How to communicate feelings assertively

➤ Identify the feeling. Watch for the signs that your body gives: do you feel a rush of adrenalin, do you feel hot, sweaty, sick, frightened or powerful?
➤ Are you on safe ground? Check that you feel safe enough to express your

feeling. If not, take steps towards temporarily controlling them. Allow yourself the time and space afterwards to release the frustration.

➤ Confront the source of the feelings. Try to identify whether you are managing immediate and direct feelings in a situation, or whether you are reacting to past hurts and stresses. If the latter, you still need to look at what is causing the feelings to surge up and how you can alleviate the problem

➤ Verbal statement. Try a simple statement: 'I am angry', 'That makes me feel very angry'. This immediately diffuses much of the tension.

Watch your non-verbal communication. Because women have few useful models for dealing with anger, we can be confused by it. Anger may make us cry, which can infuriate. It may be that we have learned to cry for sympathy, so we hope to diffuse the situation or confuse, believing people will forget the anger and concentrate instead on the sadness. Or perhaps crying was the only way we felt permitted when younger to express any deep felt emotion. Certainly, we cry with frustration and hurt. Culturally, boys and men are permitted their anger and show aggression more freely; conversely, they are not socialised to cry. Because we have odd learned behaviours, women need to watch that when they feel anger they do not smile nervously; use sarcasm or sneer, and check that tone of voice and body movements match what they say. Remember that a small, tight or little-girl voice does not carry with it the same conviction as a deeper, louder, adult one.

Using TA

Another way to manage your feelings, and to resolve conflict, is to acknowledge their history and manage the communication of them in a more conscious, adult way. Outside the therapeutic field, TA has often been used to help people remain in clear communication at an appropriate level, in counselling and consultancy, management and communications training. It is a useful tool in managing ourselves and our feelings.

In TA, 'transactions' are the flow of communication, and more specifically the unspoken psychological flow of communication (non-verbal communications) that runs in parallel. Transactions occur simultaneously at both explicit and psychological levels – *see* Section 4 for more information on this – but a common example is when we find ourselves using a caring voice with sarcastic intent. To read the real communication requires both 'surface level' and more subtle, non-verbal reading.

Using TA terminology, 'strokes' are the recognition, attention or responsiveness that one person gives another. Strokes can be positive or negative. A key idea is that people hunger for recognition, and, lacking positive strokes, will seek whatever kind they can, even if it is recognition of a negative kind. As children, we test out the strategies and behaviours that seem to get us strokes. Thus transactions can be experienced as positive or negative depending on the nature of the strokes within them. A negative transaction is preferred to no transaction at all, because of this fundamental hunger for recognition.

The nature of transactions is important to understanding communication, and how to manage communications. A simple, *reciprocal* transaction occurs when both partners are addressing the ego state the other is in. These are also called *complementary transactions* as in:

A: 'Have you been able to telephone your client?' [*adult to adult*]

B: 'Yes – I'll discuss it with you in supervision.' [*adult to adult*]

A: 'Let's skive off Monday's meeting!' [*child to child*]

B: 'Yes let's – I can't face it – what shall we do instead?' [*child to child*]

A: 'Is this your mess? I can't work amongst all these files' [*parent to child*]

B: 'Will you stop hassling me? I'll do it eventually!' [*child to parent*]

This feels very familiar: we know that communication like this can continue indefinitely, until moved into another transactionary mode.

Communication failures are typically caused by a *crossed transaction* where partners address ego states other than that which their partner is in:

A: 'Have you been able to write that report?' [*adult to adult*]

B: 'Will you stop hassling me? I'll do it eventually!' [*child to parent*]

However, if we learn to respond in adult, we stop the dynamic:

A: 'Is this your mess? I can't work among all these files.' [*parent to child*]

B: 'Sorry, yes. I'll do it now.' [*adult to adult*]

Observe how this statement puts partner B back in control, through (implicitly) acknowledging the criticism and moving on.

Another class of transaction is the more *covert* transaction, where the explicit social conversation occurs in parallel with an implicit psychological transaction. Here, again, it is important to 'stay in adult' and acknowledge the covert message, while refusing to collude. For instance:

A: 'I need you to stay late at the office with me.' [*adult words, body language indicates sexual intent – flirtatious child*]

B: 'Of course, give me a minute to phone home: I'll get the survey results out.' [*adult response to adult statement*]

If you chose to respond in child, you would smile and wink, accepting the hidden motive.

In TA theory, 'life position' refers to the general feeling about life (specifically, the unconscious feeling, as opposed to a conscious philosophical position) that colours every dyadic (i.e. person-to-person) transaction. Initially, four such life positions were proposed:

'I'm not ok, you're ok.'

'I'm not ok, you're not ok.'

'I'm ok, you're not ok.'

'I'm ok, you're ok.'

However, more recently, other life positions have been proposed that describe more significant mental health difficulties:[9] 'I'm not ok, you're ok' and 'I'm not ok, you're not ok', among others. It may be worth considering which life position you hold at present, and reflecting on how these could be applied in the following exercise.

EXERCISE 6

Match the ego state to the comment. Think about how you could bring the transaction back into Adult.

Statement	Ego states
'Oh don't worry, you did really well.'	
'Do you realise how late you always are? '	
'How do you think the presentation went?'	
'Pleeese help me, I'm really, really struggling.'	
'I'm on holiday soon, how fab is that!'	

Good, assertive responses may be:

---

9   White T. *Working with Suicidal Individuals.* Jessica Kingsley Publishers; 2011.

Statement	Ego states	Adult statement	Adult response
'Oh don't worry, you did really well.'	Nurturing parent	'This is an excellent report.'	'Yes, thank you, I wish it could have been a bit shorter but I am happy overall.'
'Do you realise how late you always are?'	Critical adult	'Let's look at what is making you late.'	'Yes, I can only apologise. We are sorting out the childcare tonight.'
'How do you think the presentation went?'	Adult	'How do you think the presentation went?'	'Fine, no problems, thanks.'
'Pleeese help me, I'm really, really struggling'	Free child	'Can you help with this a moment?'	'How can I help/ what kind of help do you need/ who can best help?'
'I've really made a mess of this – please let me try once more. please.'	Adaptive child	'I'll have another go at this and put it on your desk for the morning.'	'Ok, have another go and bring it in on Monday.'

Through doing the above work, you are taking an active role in developing your ability to examine yourself and your feelings, a prerequisite for expressing them with ease. This helps in the process of acceptance, away from shame and towards an understanding that our feelings and experiences are part of the shared human condition. We all have weaknesses and limitations, but in accepting this we can discover new ways to achieve improved self-confidence and contentment, and reach our highest potential, simply, easily and compassionately. If we acknowledge the history of our feelings and manage the communication of them in a more conscious, adult way, we find the 'adult' in ourselves, and are more likely to behave in an assertive, open minded, interested way to events and life around us.

KEY POINTS

➤ If we just work on behavioural output, there is a possibility that the change will be artificial and superficial. For real change to occur, we need to incorporate some personal awareness work. We need the conscious work to gain insight into our unconscious emotions and drives.

➤ We need to gain awareness and understanding of our feelings, how we operate and are seen by others, and identify how some of our usually unquestioned thoughts, behaviours and immediate responses are possibly dysfunctional, unrealistic or unhelpful.

➤ The ability to have empathy for difference, to be open to diversity, to work hard at noticing difference, is crucial to the work of being assertive.

➤ Feelings are part of the human condition, not personal, isolating or shameful. We need to face our own difficulties with compassion.

➤ One key is the ability to engage your cognition and intellect and rely less on feeling and more on rational thought. Thus it is important to verbalise feelings.

➤ To help us identify how we feel, use all the senses as well as our thoughts and emotions. Try to identify the physical feeling that goes with the emotion.

➤ Some of our feelings are generated by the re-stimulation of old 'scripts', old and familiar ways of being in the world. We need to find the 'adult' in ourselves, and behave instead in an open-minded, but logical, interested way to events and life around us.

➤ Although people can argue with your logic, they cannot deny or dismiss your feelings. You have a right to them.

➤ Feelings often conflict with what we think is rational. If your present reaction seems inappropriate, you could be responding to something unresolved from your past.

➤ We need to be able to make choices in our lives. If this need is blocked, we experience frustration, helplessness, irritation, anger. If the need if fulfilled, we feel powerful, enthused and energised.

➤ We need to feel understood. If this need is satisfied, we feel secure, safe and valued.

➤ Feelings are powerful, and negative feelings provoke fear. If you can, stay with and verbalise feelings rather than avoiding them.

➤ Anger can be a very motivating force: it can motivate us to change things; it gives us the impetus to move direction in life or take up challenges; it can be vigorous, creative and determined. If we understand and express anger assertively, we act to revoke those feelings of resentment and powerlessness and create change in our lives.

FURTHER READING

Berne E. *Games People Play: the psychology of human relationships*. Penguin; 2010.

Germer CK. *The Mindful Path to Self-Compassion: freeing yourself from destructive thoughts and emotions*. The Guilford Press; 2009.

Gilbert P. *Compassion Focused Therapy: distinctive features (CBT distinctive features)*. Routledge; 2010.

Lindenfield G. *Assert Yourself: a self-help assertiveness programme for men and women*. Thorsons; 1992.

CHAPTER 6

Dealing with criticism

'People who demand perfection from themselves, or expect approval from significant others, can often take criticism badly …'[1]

If you are the kind of person who dreads appraisals and takes any criticism, however well meant, very personally, this chapter is for you. It is usual to feel prickly and defensive when criticised, but not usual to feel devastated. If you take criticism very seriously, you are more likely to translate the comments into feelings of generalised unworthiness. These feelings can overwhelm, preventing a rational, adult response. An assertive response is only a tool, and although it can be learnt, it does not replace the need for you to investigate the reasons you respond as you do. It is only through looking at and understanding these reasons, however painful, that we can begin to understand ourselves and respond authentically, not reactively. It may help to consider that constructive criticism can help us to understand ourselves better, and improve our work performance and relationships. Criticism is something we all experience from time to time.

The assertive person has to be open to, and be able to give and receive, criticism honestly and fairly. In this chapter we look at some of the best ways to accept criticism: by assessing it and exposing it as direct, indirect or manipulative; and we also look at some of the ways to give criticism skilfully, cleanly and fairly, without guise.

Preparation is crucial, hence the work on feelings. Assertive people are not frightened of criticism because they are well prepared for it and know that it can be useful to all parties concerned.[2] Prepare yourself to know your likely reactions by building up some self-awareness. Once you have an idea of why you are feeling tearful, angry or defensive, you will be more prepared to tolerate these ambiguous or difficult feelings. From this position, you can act more clearly. You will be more able to accept criticism from others, and also be able to give it yourself.

---

1   Willson R, Branch R. *Cognitive Behaviour Therapy for Dummies*. John Wiley & Sons; 2006. pp. 3, 13, 186.
2   Lindenfield G. *Assert Yourself: simple steps to getting what you want*. Thorsons; 2001.

DEALING WITH CRITICISM

You will need to learn to distinguish between criticisms, which are valid, invalid or simply a 'put-down'.

Valid criticisms are those that you know are legitimate. Only you know if you truly are an impatient person, or always late, or change your mind a lot, so if people accuse you of these things and you know they do apply, learn to accept the comment graciously rather than getting defensive. If you feel you still need to work on self-awareness, try this exercise.

EXERCISE 1

Johari Window[3] is commonly used as a model for mapping personality aware-ness. By describing yourself from a fixed list of adjectives, then asking your friends and colleagues to describe you from the same list, a grid of overlap and difference can be built up.

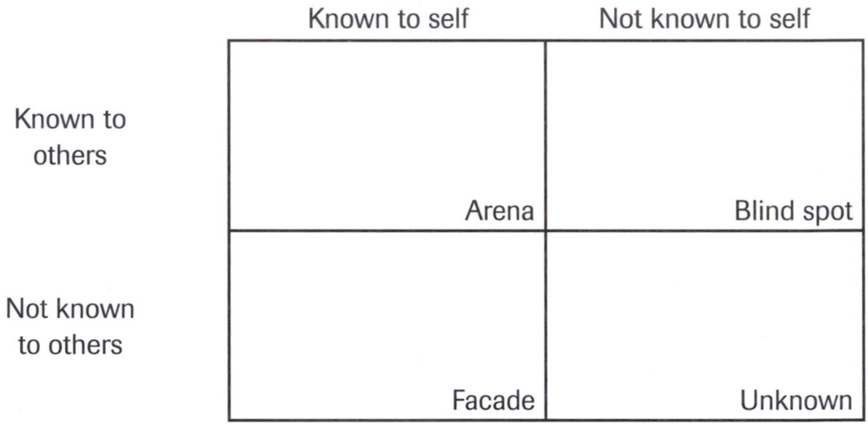

	Known to self	Not known to self
Known to others	Arena	Blind spot
Not known to others	Facade	Unknown

Figure 6.1 The Johari Window

Arena: this represents traits of the subjects that both they and their peers are aware of.

Facade: adjectives selected only by subjects, but not by any of their peers, are placed here, representing information about them their peers are unaware of.

Blind spot: adjectives selected only by peers are placed here. These represent information that the subject is not aware of, but others are.

Unknown: adjectives that were not selected by either subjects or their peers are placed here, representing behaviours that were not recognised by anyone participating.

---

3 Luft J, Ingham H. The Johari Window, a graphic model of interpersonal awareness. *Proceedings of the Western Training Laboratory in Group Development.* Los Angeles: UCLA; 1950.

To get started, select from the following words that you feel best describe you:

able	accepting	adaptable	bold	brave
calm	caring	cheerful	clever	complex
confident	dependable	dignified	energetic	extroverted
friendly	giving	happy	helpful	idealistic
independent	ingenious	intelligent	introverted	kind
knowledgeable	logical	loving	mature	modest
nervous	observant	organised	patient	powerful
proud	quiet	reflective	relaxed	religious
responsive	searching	self-assertive	self-conscious	sensible
sentimental	shy	silly	spontaneous	sympathetic
tense	trustworthy	warm	wise	witty

EXERCISE 2

Personal Effectiveness Scale (PES)[4]

This online scale comprises three factors: self-disclosure, openness to feedback and perceptiveness. Self-disclosure score is plotted horizontally, whereas the openness to feedback score is plotted vertically. The window formed naturally displays the sizes of the open, hidden, blind spot and unknown areas, giving a perspective into the individual's personality.

EXERCISE 3

Dream Johari Window

The Dream Johari Window represents what an individual wants his or her personality to be like. The sizes of the areas in the Dream Window may be different from the sizes of the same areas in the current Window. An individual with a Dream Window identical to the current window may have higher self-awareness. The perceptiveness score from the PES indicates how likely it is for the individual to achieve the Dream Window. For example, a high score on the PES indicates a higher possibility of transition.

Use the knowledge gained from these exercises to judge for yourself whether criticism aimed at you are valid or invalid. When managing *valid criticisms*, we need to learn to listen well to what people are saying. There may be times when we need to accept the truth. If you cannot accept a criticism instantly, no

---

4   www.empiindia.com/portal/safi/index.php?pid=udaipareek (accessed April 2013).

matter – think about what was said and return to it another time. It may well be that whatever is being said is unpalatable, certainly it may be something about yourself you do not want to hear or accept. Ask yourself if there is some truth in the criticism.

➤ Do you have a tendency to bully, to use your position to get what you want at the expense of others?

➤ Do you sometimes feel inadequate so you assert yourself unnecessarily and cause others to feel small or powerless as a consequence?

➤ Are you judgmental (it feels easier to criticise and blame others rather than look inside at your own failings and weaknesses)?

If you feel defensive and angry, there is probably some truth in what others are saying.

Invalid criticisms are those that you know within yourself to be clearly untrue, and can be rejected as such.

➤ They are often global statements or accusations such as: 'You're so mean/lazy/unsociable.'

➤ If they feel completely unfair and incorrect, then say so.

➤ These comments are more likely to be said in anger, and reflect the other person's feelings more than your own.

Manipulative criticisms lead you to feel 'put-down' in some way; someone is trying to score a point using you as the bait.

➤ These comments are made by people who probably do not feel good about themselves, and need to make others feel bad in order to feel better themselves (in TA terms, 'I'm not ok, you're not ok').

➤ These types of comments look like a compliment or casual comment on the surface, but in fact on reflection are something more unpleasant. They are the veiled comments that make you feel angry or hurt.

➤ If you confront the person and venture to say that their comment hurt you, you may be met with denial: 'Oh, I didn't mean it like that!' They are the sorts of remark used to create a reaction.

An example of an effective response to this sort of situation is given below.

Sarah is a social work manager running a busy service. She has had the decorators in her room for over four days and the place has been in chaos. Work carried on as usual, meetings were held, and visitors were seen, in an area cordoned off for the purpose. It was the end of the fourth day and Sarah was just about to lock up when one of the decorators, who was packing up, turned to her, saying:

'Of course I had a run in with one of you lot years ago, trying to get a social worker to see my brother, but it didn't help. I think you managers are all very well but the way the council is going I reckon they'd be better off spending all that money on social workers instead of frittering it away on things that don't do much good. Seems to me the money could be better spent on getting those social workers out to see people instead of getting them to push paper all the time. No offence to you, love, but really, don't you think you'd be better off helping out in reception instead of swanking around up here?'

Sarah could respond by going into a long diatribe or justification for her service; proving to him that any big organisation needed someone to take charge; detailing the chronic underfunding of social services overall. Instead, she sees this situation for what it is – someone with a personal grudge to bear and an outsiders' knowledge of the service gained through the media. She quickly decides that she does not want to be drawn into a lengthy, defensive, discussion so says:

'Derek, I know you'd like to chat but I've had a long day and I'm tired. I'm going to lock up now. Can you let yourself out?'

She thus understands his need to offload, but explains how she feels, ignores the bait and terminates the conversation by asking an unrelated question.

Put-downs are designed to make you feel small. They can be subtly disguised as social niceties or jokes. If you respond with sarcasm, it may be viewed as indirect aggression: it will certainly be more competitive than constructive. Instead, invest your energy in asserting your own needs, or in taking some positive action to get what you want. In responding to put-downs, aim to protect your rights and self-esteem by letting the other person know that you recognise the hidden message, thus putting a quick stop to the behaviour.

How to deal with frequently used indirect criticisms

In the following scenario, the speaker is asking her manager if it is possible to implement a new cost-saving idea. Whenever I have used the following responses it is because I have felt tired, stressed, insecure or unsure of my authority and position. The assertive respondent needs to recognise this and such indirect communication needs dealing with firmly and honestly. Make it the speaker's problem, not yours. Expose the dishonesty by taking the speaker at their word, bringing the transaction back into adult.

'If this were up to me, I'd agree to it, but …'

➤ Find out who is responsible.
➤ Tell them about another manager who has supported you.

➤ Get more information about the decision maker mentioned that you can use in your favour.

> 'This is a lot more complex than it looks.'

➤ Tease out and deal with the stated complexities.
➤ Ask for a quick summary of the issues.
➤ Focus on the key elements.
➤ Use to develop a common understanding of the issue.

> 'I don't think there is time to take your ideas on board.'

➤ Ask them to explain why the deadline is so tight.
➤ Would there ever have been time for your input, and if not, why not?
➤ Get them to accept your ideas in principle, finding ways to change the time frame.

> 'If you'd done this yourself you would know.'

➤ Move the issue onto common ground so you can talk in equal terms.
➤ Acknowledge the feelings: 'I do respect your experience but I'd like to find a way of understanding your perspective on this.'

> 'I don't think you need worry yourself about this.'

➤ Say you would find it really valuable if you could understand the finer points.
➤ Stress how much your understanding can help them.

> 'There are other agendas you don't know about.'

➤ Establish your legitimate interest in the matter.
➤ Get that accepted.
➤ Ask the speaker to be more specific.

Very often racist or sexist humour is disguised indirect criticism, and one of the best ways to deal with this is take it at face value, literally. If someone cracks a joke which makes you feel uncomfortable, expose it, and their motives, by admitting you do not understand and asking them to explain?

> 'I don't get why it would be funny for a non-English talker to ask that?'

> 'Can you explain why the woman would …?'

Or an intake of breath – 'That's difficult' – to indicate you find it problematic or hurtful.

This kind of pragmatic response forces the speaker to recognise the unpleasantness of his or her joke: they have to face the embarrassment of explaining their frankly difficult and oppressive 'humour', not you.

You can use this approach to expose other kinds of indirect or direct criticism. When you are faced with someone who appears to blame or threaten you try the following.

➤ **Indirect blame:** response: 'I really respect you, but it is not my cross to bear that you feel this/have these [*particular issues*].'

➤ **Threat:** 'You said you would sort this.' Response: offer a choice: 'Yes I did, and I did my best, but I can't be responsible for the whole job here.'

What is your reaction to criticism?

Very few people are truly invulnerable to criticism and most of us would admit to one of the following reactions. Do you respond non-assertively by avoiding the person who is criticising you? If your ego is weak or fragile, or if you are acting with little awareness of yourself and your feelings, you are more likely to respond with anger. Or do you avoid criticism by keeping quiet, ingratiating yourself to others; do you stay in a position of less authority or responsibility that you are capable of? This may be a valid option in intolerable circumstances: to take yourself out of a difficult situation, but if you regularly avoid confrontation:

➤ this passive behaviour can irritate others

➤ it does not do you justice in your ability to deal with life

➤ it does not enhance self-development

➤ it becomes easy to accept and absorb the criticism

➤ avoidance decreases your self-esteem and does not enhance your confidence

➤ it damages you in the long term by building up anger and resentment.

Assertive behaviour

Here are some examples of how assertiveness experts would recommend you deal with criticism, using the techniques developed by Anne Dickson.[5]

Agree

This is a useful technique to use with hostile or constructive criticism. Check first if the criticism applies to you and, if it is valid and legitimate, thank your critic for the feedback.

---

5   Dickson A, Charlesworth K. *A Woman in Your Own Right*. Quartet; 1982.

➤ Agree. 'Yes, I am very untidy', 'Yes, I agree, it was stupid of me to respond to him so aggressively'. In agreeing you disarm your critic if they are using the criticism as hostile bait and you develop self-acceptance.

➤ Be honest. If it is a trait you rather like in yourself, say so. If someone criticised you for being a perfectionist, you could respond by saying: 'Yes, I am a perfectionist, and I know that sometimes I expect too much from the staff, but I think that it's a good trait and I'm not prepared to lower my standards.'

➤ If someone criticises you in an area that you are trying to improve, try: 'Yes, I know I'm being a bit diffident, I'm finding it difficult to make up my mind on this one. I'm sorry if it's a bit irritating, but I am trying to learn to be more concise. I am improving, but I need time.'

Deny it

If the criticism is totally invalid, do not accept it at all, but say with conviction: 'That's completely untrue/unfair/unjust. I am not going to accept that.' Be certain, do not apologise or doubt.

Accept with reservation

Ask for specification if you feel the criticism is global or unjust. This makes it more manageable. If someone accuses you of *always* being late and you feel this is untrue, you could say: 'No, I don't accept that I'm always late. I was late today, and I know that I arrived late for that meeting last month, but as a rule I am on time.' Accept the part of the criticism that is valid, but do not take on board the sort of sweeping generalisation that, if accepted, could gradually lower your self-esteem. Calmly acknowledge that there may be some truth in what is being said. Make your own assessment of the situation: 'Yes I was late this morning. Possibly I am not as committed to work at the moment as I usually am. Can we talk about this?'

Accepting criticism is very powerful. It reinforces the idea that you alone have the right to act as a judge of your own behaviour and refuses to reward the critic who is trying to 'put you down'. It acknowledges there is some truth in their statement and also encourages the critic to learn to be more specific with their criticisms.

Ask for examples

Sometimes you feel that a criticism has a grain of truth in it, or you feel uncertain if your critic is manipulating you. This technique gives you time to think, and enables you to hear a little more about what the other person is trying to tell you. If the criticism is constructive, you will be able to use that information to learn. You can use this technique to prompt criticism – because you are initiating it, you are able to operate from a position of strength.

Some examples of this are as follows.

➤ 'In what ways do you think I am lazy?'
➤ 'You say that you are concerned that I am too critical in my dealings with patients. Can you give me some examples?'
➤ 'Are you saying that you are dissatisfied with the quality of my work?'
➤ 'Do you find me a bit too pushy at times?'
➤ 'Are you angry that I'm late?'

When you invite criticism, you are opening up a frank and truthful exchange of feelings. This is a powerful way of enabling someone to feel secure enough to express negative feelings to you, and also helps you to feel secure enough to listen to what is being said. Here are some of the examples Anne Dickson[6] uses to illustrate this.

➤ 'I've been very preoccupied lately. Do you find this frustrating?'
➤ 'I talk a lot when I'm anxious. Does this irritate you?'
➤ 'I know I'm inconsistent. Does it drive you up the wall?'

Some advantages of this approach are that:
➤ when you invite criticism, you are in a much stronger position to handle it
➤ when you choose when you are going to ask, you are back in control of the situation
➤ the more often you survive hearing something you do not like about yourself, the easier it will be to deal with criticism
➤ you begin to be able to use the criticism wisely, to judge for yourself what is said and to use the opportunity to learn.

Much criticism is given out of genuine respect and kindness, with the wish to reach out and help, to improve communication and deepen understanding. It can demonstrate someone's clear regard for you.

GIVING CRITICISM

If you need honesty and openly to discuss another colleague's work, or talk with a parent about how they are managing a situation badly, or share your concerns with a patient or client about some aspect of their behaviour, you need to follow some key rules. You need to take the initiative, so be well prepared and work in a space where you will not be disturbed. Allow the other person time to prepare. Act quickly, being very specific about the problem, avoiding

---

6   Dickson, Charlesworth, note 5 above.

indirect attack and blame (never make assumptions about why people behave as they do: ask). Talk about and take responsibility for your own feelings, and demonstrate that you understand and empathise with their position. Spell out the consequences of their behaviour and be prepared to compromise. Be calm, phrase positively and always end on a positive note.

SUMMARY

➤ Allow the other person *time to prepare*; give some indication of the matter you wish to discuss.

➤ *Act quickly.* If you defer and wait until the next time the problem arises, your feelings about the issue will, if anything, be stronger, and hence less controllable.

➤ Set aside time to talk about the issue in a place where you will *not be disturbed*. Give yourself plenty of time to plan what you are going to say beforehand.

➤ *Be specific.* Instead of dropping vague hints that you are irritated by poor time keepers, confront the issue: 'Matt, we feel frustrated when you are late. Could you try and arrive by 4 o'clock next time?'

➤ Be prepared to *compromise*: 'If this is difficult for you maybe we could all discuss starting the meeting later ...'

➤ *Express how you feel* about the behaviour, and the effect it has on you, the organisation or the patients. Take responsibility for your feelings: 'I feel angry and hurt when ...'

➤ *Avoid direct attack and blame* – whether in the form of 'You're so immature' or 'You should be more ...'. This will always be unsolicited, unwanted advice. Global, judgemental or generalised statements about someone's behaviour are basically attacks on their personality. Avoid labels or stereotypes – for example: 'You're such a wimp', 'That's a typical female response'. Again, state how you feel, specifically, about the one item of behaviour you want changed.

➤ *Do not assume* you know what motivates other people – you may be mistaken. Avoid analysis such as: 'She must have known how much that would hurt' – it is impossible to interpret other peoples' behaviour.

➤ *Spell out the consequences.* These may be positive: 'I will feel much less strained if you could be on time' or 'I feel resentful when you leave all the paperwork to me. I know you don't like doing it but I would like to share the load more equally. That would leave both of us more time for our clinic work'.

If the consequences are negative, spell them out too. Clarity helps people in their decision making. Chose the level you want: 'I would feel much happier if ...', or 'If there is no change, I will have no option but to leave'.

If the change you anticipate or hope for does not come about, be prepared to ride the consequences. Remember that we can always change our behaviour, but we cannot expect others to change theirs, however much we want them too. You can ask, but you may not get what you want.

➤ View the other person *as an equal*. If you do take the initiative to confront, remember that you in turn may be confronted.

➤ *Take responsibility*. Invariably, people are surprised, and often shocked, when you mention that part of their behaviour has had such an effect on you, so do take responsibility for not mentioning it before:

> 'I'm sorry that I didn't make myself clear before.'

> 'I take full blame: you weren't to know.'

> 'I should have mentioned it before, but I didn't feel able.'

> 'I should have sorted it out and been direct but I was frightened of your reaction.'

➤ *Take the initiative*. Even if you have taken the initiative to confront, use the opportunity to invite criticism: 'I should have mentioned this before, I expect I've surprised/ upset/ angered you.'

➤ *Empathise*. Understand the other person's position. Start with something on the lines of: 'I realize that what I have to say will be upsetting …'

➤ *Keep calm*. Make sure that you keep your voice level and avoid using threatening gestures.

➤ *Phrase and reinforce positively*. 'It would be better if you talked more loudly' gives someone the hope of being both better heard and better regarded if they make that change. Saying the same thing negatively, 'It would be better if you did not talk so quietly', can leave the person concentrating on their sense of failure rather than wanting to improve

➤ *End on a positive note*. Find a remark to balance the interaction, to give some indication that you value the other person and are not only seeing the negative: 'I'm grateful to you for listening' or 'I'm glad that we've aired this'. If you wish, you may like to add a positive statement about the other person: 'I do hope that my having said this will not adversely affect our relationship. I've always found you especially easy to talk too, and I do value the way we work so well together.' Or you may prefer to end the conversation with a positive consequence; something on the lines of: 'I'm glad that we've cleared the air. Now I feel that I'll be more relaxed in your company.' Be honest and true to yourself, mean what you say.

Giving and receiving compliments

We do not always find it easy to give or receive compliments, given as women we have been socialised to be diffident and not to 'show off', reveal, display or exhibit the best of ourselves intellectually; nor do we always feel comfortable acting competitively with our peers or others. We thus find it harder to take the power and praise others; we use defeatist self-talk ('What right have I got …', 'They must think I think a lot about myself', 'Who am I …'). However, part of being assertive is to challenge yourself, and to act powerfully and strongly. You have every right to praise, admire and demonstrate respect for other people's behaviour, and, if you are a manager or supervisor, it will be a big part of your job, both formally in appraisal and informally, to demonstrate kindly observation of someone's abilities. In observing 'good' behaviour, or a job well done, you need to be both sincere and specific.

Accepting compliments is also hard for women. Men, with their more competitive nature and, often, bigger ego, find it easier to accept compliments. When accepting compliments, do not be diffident. Pause, notice the praise and then simply agree! Thank the person praising you, do not reject, deny or minimise. Try a simple 'Thank you' without a rider, a 'But'. The pause may help you to identify backhanded comments, and if so, to deal with them as an invalid criticism. Challenge some of the fixed, negative ideas you have about yourself by making a further list of your good and bad points. This will help you to understand yourself and your behaviour more, to be able to identify a true compliment and to deal with criticism more constructively.

EXERCISE 4

Identify and list some criticisms you have received from:

Parents	
Friends	
Partners	
Children	
Employers	
Employees	

Are these criticisms fair or not?

EXERCISE 5

Make a table and write down five unfair criticisms about yourself in the left column. On the right, write down five fair criticisms.

	Unfair	Fair
1		
2		
3		
4		
5		

With a partner, pair up and swap lists. Each person reads out items at random from the lists to his or her partner, who has to respond appropriately, for example:

> 'I feel that is an unfair criticism, I will not accept that. Can you give me an example of when I am mean …'

or

> 'I accept that criticism. I do tend to be bossy, and I'm trying to stop it.'

EXERCISE 6

With a friend, each writes down 10 valid criticisms, 10 that you consider invalid (remember, you may need to revise these later!) and 10 things that you like about yourself. Be specific. Instead of using words like 'good', 'bad' or 'nice' try 'excellent', 'incompetent', 'friendly'. Here is part of my list:

Valid

I talk too much, and interrupt
I'm too bossy
I'm impatient
I'm a perfectionist

Invalid

I'm lazy
I'm disorganised
I'm too critical
I'm unsociable

Personal positives

I'm friendly
I'm competent in my job
I can put people at their ease

Swap lists. Each person reads out items at random from the list to his or her partner, beginning with that person's name, for example: 'Olivia, you're too bossy.' The partner has to respond appropriately, using the skills outlined above, for example:

> 'Yes, I accept that I am bossy. Part of my job is to tell people what to do.'

> 'I feel that is an unfair criticism. I will not accept that I am disorganised. Can you give me an example?'

> 'Thank you. I'm proud of the work I do here.' [*when given a compliment that you are good at your job*]

EXERCISE 7

Things I do badly

Take it in turns to say the thing you do most badly for example: 'I am very bad at keeping time.'

In the next round, each of you says the thing that other people tell them thy do well for example: 'People say I'm a good listener.' In the next round, stand up and tell your partner about the thing that you do well. Ham it up, exaggerate it and show off: 'I'm the world champion at …'

EXERCISE 8

Look honestly at those aspects of your behaviour that you suspect irritate, disappoint or anger others. Be honest with yourself. Write down these aspects and what you could say to those people if you were to use the skills of negative assertion and negative enquiry.

Expect and accept compliments graciously. Over one week, make a note of how many compliments you have given, taken or rejected. Set yourself a goal to note and praise a colleague or a client's behaviour more frequently. Over the following weeks, aim to give one extra compliment away each day and note how you felt and how each gesture was received.

KEY POINTS

➤ Criticism is something we all experience from time to time. The assertive person has to be open to, and be able to give and receive, criticism honestly and fairly.

➤ Very few people are truly invulnerable to criticism. If you take criticism very seriously, you are more likely to translate the comments into feelings of generalised unworthiness. If so, investigate the reasons why you respond as you do. Once you have an idea of why you are feeling tearful, angry or defensive, you will be more prepared to tolerate these ambiguous or difficult feelings. From this position, you can act more clearly. You will be more able to accept criticism from others, and also be able to give it yourself.

➤ Distinguish between criticisms which are valid, invalid or simply a 'put-down'.

➤ Ask yourself if there is some truth in the criticism, as if patently untrue it can be rejected. Agree with valid criticism, deny invalid criticism, or ask for specification and examples, and invite criticism to double check.

➤ Confront manipulative criticism or 'jokes' you feel uncomfortable with. Get your communication partner back into 'adult': expose it; get more information; develop a common understanding of the issue; ask them to explain; acknowledge the feelings.

➤ You may avoid criticism by keeping quiet or ingratiating yourself with others; this may be a valid option in intolerable circumstances, but if you regularly avoid confrontation it becomes easy to accept and absorb the criticism, and this decreases your self-esteem.

Giving criticism

When giving criticism:

➤ set the scene
➤ act quickly
➤ be specific
➤ do not judge
➤ describe your feelings
➤ be aware of the consequences, both negative and positive
➤ take responsibility
➤ ask for feedback
➤ empathise
➤ keep calm
➤ use the 'stuck record' technique
➤ phrase positively
➤ end on a positive note.

Receiving criticism

Distinguish between:
➤ valid – if valid, agree
➤ invalid – if invalid, reject, part accept, deny or ask for more information
➤ manipulative – if manipulative, deflect or ignore.

Compliments

When giving compliments:

➤ be sincere
➤ be specific.

When accepting compliments:
➤ agree
➤ give thanks
➤ do not reject, deny or minimise – try: 'Thank you', not 'But I laugh like a hyena!'
➤ identify backhanders and deal with them as invalid criticisms
➤ challenge some of the fixed, negative ideas you have about yourself – if any are negative, swap them for a positive.

CHAPTER 7

Making and refusing requests

SAYING 'NO'

Consider the following. Do you instantly respond with a 'yes' if you are asked favour at home or at work? Are you setting yourself up to be a super-woman/manager/doctor/therapist/nurse? Or do you feel comfortable refusing requests, and can you live with the guilt that may follow?

We have already discussed how women especially find it easy to get caught up in this scenario as culturally, women are taught to be selfless and caring. They are taught readily to give up their own needs in order that someone else feels comfortable. They are taught, both overtly and subtly, that their own needs should come last. This behaviour can, of course, have a pay-off: by being seen to 'do it all' and cope, women claw back some of the power that is unevenly distributed between the sexes. We struggle to delegate as it feels easier, and better, to do it ourselves. Especially at home, offers of help are withdrawn, and the power is regained. We have the knowledge, authority and ability – at home we rule. Perhaps in the short term, but others then suffer from not learning from the experience, and those who fail to delegate can burn out with overwork.

It takes great effort to relinquish some of that power. Making the choice to do so can be very freeing, but it can also cause some internal conflict, as the adult woman is taking a stand against the child within her, and that new role takes time to nurture and grow. Women are socialised to be compliant, to win approval. It can be very difficult to throw off that innate dependence and continuing need for (parental) approval, but it is not impossible. When we become an adult, we can, and do, make our own choices in life – by saying 'no' for ourselves we are rejecting the underlying need to be liked; we chose for ourselves. In delegating, we reap new rewards and gain a different power that is non-manipulative. We learn more about the power of equality, of real choice. We learn to be assertive and to share.

In this chapter, we explore some of these differences and their impact on the ways men and women communicate, together and with each other, and how this affects our ability to be assertive. Later chapters give a more detailed and focused look at language and non-verbal behaviour in relation to the skill being taught.

Language enables us to communicate in many different ways, for many different purposes. We do not always mean what we say.[1] When we say 'yes', we do not always mean it: it is politeness that dictates that we do not say 'no'. We can speak the same word or sentence with an altogether different meaning, when the meaning is in the tone of voice, the stress, pausing, intonation and context. The way the sentence is phrased, the syntax – word order – will also have an impact. Gender and culture differences mean that things said one way are interpreted differently by others. Paralinguistics is a term for the study of how things are said and how this affects the meaning of what is said. It looks at language purposes, some of the hidden meanings, expectations and assumptions in our language, some of the ways we communicate, and includes the study of how men and women's discourse differs. Think of all the different we can say 'really', or any word or sentence – with affirmation, ridicule, sarcasm, uncertainty, confidence or acceptance. The meaning is in the tone of voice, the stress, pausing, intonation and context (for more on language and non-verbal behaviour, *see* Section 4). The word 'no' can thus be said in different ways (happily, laughing, begrudgingly, sarcastically) depending on the meaning you wish to imply.

Beneath spoken language there are always hidden meanings. There is an unstated but 'heard' ranking/power dynamic that plays out. Compliments are always given by those of higher rank to those of lower rank, and talk/subject matter is always initiated by the higher ranking. There are differences in the way men and women vie for power, for status and connection.

Early feminists such as Deborah Tannen[2] acknowledged that both genders have different repertoires and we have different expectations about how men and women present, their expectations, their core beliefs. It is therefore hard for women to say 'no', and instead we tend to 'soften' it by saying: 'Is it alright if ...', 'Do you mind if ...', 'Can I charge you for (less) than the two hours?'.

There is also a cultural issue for us here in the West. Politeness dictates that we do not say 'no'. In this context, culturally, it is also unacceptable to say 'no' to a request for a favour from a significant other in our life, someone important or superior to us: friend, family member or manager ('Can can I borrow your car?', 'Will you babysit for me tonight?', 'Can you cover the phones

---

1 Townsend J. Paralinguistics: it's not what you say it's the way that you say it. *Management Decision*. 1988; **26**(3): 26–40. Crystal D. Prosody and paralinguistic correlates of social categories. In: Gardener E, editor. *Social Anthropology and Language*. Tavistock; 1971. pp. 185–206.

2 Tannen D. *Talking Voices: repetition, dialogue, and imagery in conversational discourse*. Cambridge University Press; 2007. Tannen D. *You Just Don't Understand: women and men in conversation*. New ed. Virago; 1992. Tannen D. *Talking from 9 to 5: women and men at work*. Avon; 1994. Tannen D. *Gender and Discourse*. Oxford University Press; 1996.

for half an hour?') can be exceptionally difficult to refuse. There is a recognised power balance that makes refusal difficult – it is easy to refuse your child a sweet because you hold the power, less easy to refuse your superior or parent; there are friendship allegiances, there are issues of passivity and wanting to be accepted, liked.

Consider some of the work situations in which it is difficult to make a refusal.

➤ A commissioning manager is pressing you for some information that is confidential to your practice.

➤ You are seeing a patient to talk through a complaint. The conversation drifts away from the subject in hand towards another problem they have. You feel sorry for the patient and flattered that you are being asked for advice. It becomes increasingly hard to end the conversation.

➤ You are approached and asked if you could give a lift home to the senior partner's two children, who live near to you, but in fact not in the direction you usually take. You are pressed for time as you have an evening commitment.

➤ You are invited to a colleague's retirement party on an evening that clashes with your child's open evening at school.

Refer back to Chapter 2 on women at work to remind yourself how, culturally, these situations are so hard for us to deal with. Language enables us to communicate in many different ways, for many different purposes. Feminists acknowledge that both genders have different repertoires and we have different expectations about how men and women present, their expectations, their core beliefs.

EXERCISE 1

Here is a list of stereotypical male and female characteristics. Which of these do you consider male and which are female? Mark each with a score from 1 to 10, with 10 being strongly female:

➤ indirectness
➤ interrupting frequently
➤ happy with silence
➤ volubility
➤ directness/honesty
➤ gossip
➤ asking questions to understand the other person
➤ raising new topics of interest to self
➤ wanting to mend it all or problem solve
➤ conflict and verbal aggression

➤ raising topics of interest to listener
➤ high confidence
➤ frequent apologies
➤ high aggression
➤ topic cohesion – keeping to topic
➤ asking lots of questions to gain information
➤ believing you have got it wrong
➤ believing the other person has got it wrong.

Now look at those you have given a high female count to. It is hard to give a firm and clear 'no'; when you have been socialised to be more compliant, to apologise, to have lower confidence in yourself and your abilities and rights. As a woman, one way you can regain some power, and learn to stand up for yourself and your needs, is to take a critical look at how you present as a woman. Does your presentation and body language 'mark' you as someone without much power and authority? If you are unhappy with this, make a conscious decision to present yourself more strongly. Check your body language: make sure you look the person in the eye as you say 'no', or try moving away or making a 'no' hand movement if the 'no' is final and blunt. Check that you are not smiling apologetically as you talk; maintain firm eye contact; sit or stand upright; and keep your voice steady and clear.

To help you in this process, start to unpick what you see about you – how others present themselves. Look for signs of dominance and submission in people's verbal and non-verbal behaviour, looking at both 'gross' and 'fine' features, gross being large body movements, sitting, standing, arm crossing; 'fine' being eye movements, facial expressions, tone of voice, etc.

EXERCISE 2

Listen to and watch people. Compare DVD/radio footage/observe them on public transport. Soaps and dramas make excellent observation platforms, because the behaviours are so extreme and stereotypical. Make a rough count of your observations. Make a mental note of the behaviours you see about you, on a continuum of submissive/passive and confident/aggressive. Make a note of what you observe. Who crosses their legs, smiles most frequently? Who takes up seats in the tube, unapologetically? Who stares, challenges? Features to look for include:
➤ body space/body positioning
➤ facial expressions and use of gesture, head positioning – head tilt, etc.
➤ who takes up the most verbal space when men and women are together
➤ in which situations (compare meetings at work with the pub)
➤ intonation.

	Body space/ dominance	Use of gesture	Facial expressions	'Air time'
Men				
Women				

Take an honest look at how you present: the more complicated the clothes, jewellery, accessories and make-up you wear, the more female your presentation, and possibly the less seriously you will be taken professionally. If you feel this is the case, and if you want to, tone it down a fraction, remembering that within your choice of image it is still possible to show strength of character and keep your power with words and body language. Lower the pitch of your voice, increase the volume and increase your assertiveness rating.

Having acknowledged that it is difficult, but not impossible, for women to move out of the compassion trap, let us look at some of the common misconceptions about saying 'no'.

'Saying "no" directly is rude and blunt'

Because we are unused to saying 'no' without padding or excuses, we tend to feel that it is impolite, but a 'no' can be said politely, and with respect.
➤ Take responsibility for your decision.
➤ Allow the other person space to express their feelings.
➤ Practice saying 'no' clearly and directly, without padding, frills or apology.
➤ Do not elaborate, offer excuses or explanation – you do not need to.
➤ Take responsibility for saying 'no', rather than blaming someone else.
➤ Acknowledge their problem, but stay with your answer – 'no'.

'I can see your predicament, but I can't help you.'

'I know that it will be difficult for you to find someone else for the evening, but no, I can't help you out tonight.'

'Saying "no" is selfish, uncaring and mean'

By saying 'no', you are being clear about your own wishes and needs, and people will respect you for this honesty. When someone asks you to do something, you do not have to respond. Remind yourself when you last asked someone for a favour, or to spend time with you on a project, or to provide cover for you, and they refused. No doubt you accepted their refusal without question. Allow yourself the same freedom and respect that you give others.

➤ Your own needs are important.
➤ Your own needs are no more or less important than anyone else's, but of equal import.
➤ Say 'no' more frequently and you can begin to balance your own needs with that of other people.

This is not self-preoccupation or narcissism, but a description of balanced care, extended with the same concern to self as others. In saying 'no' you are setting new limits for yourself; you are giving yourself adequate time to rest and replenish your energy to enable you to make more active choices on how you spend your time. People rarely admire or respect someone who thinks so little of herself that she never gives herself time. Remember that when intent on being selfless, we easily become overstretched and exhausted by our responsibilities – at great cost to our physical and mental well-being.

'People won't like me if I say "no"'

Will people really think you selfish or greedy if you say 'no'? In fact, the reverse is often true: people respect you for being clear about your own limitations. And because you are more in control of yourself and your own time, you respect yourself more, too. When you acknowledge any negative feelings that you feel the other person has about your refusal, there should be no reason for their dislike. An assertive 'no' should leave both parties feeling comfortable. If we suppress a lot of our negative feelings in order to gain love and respect, we deny that we have any needs. We then do all that is asked of us but end up saying 'no' indirectly, in a begrudging way.

'Saying "no" will cause others to take offence. It will make them feel rejected and hurt'

You are refusing the *request* not the *person* when you say 'no'. If you anticipate that your 'no' will be hurtful in some way, remember to acknowledge that.

'Disagreement and conflict are a disaster and must be avoided at all costs'

➤ Not so. Everyone we meet is unique and likely to hold different views.
➤ It can be very refreshing, intellectually and emotionally, to discuss these differences.
➤ Conflict can be painful, but we learn through its resolution.

Being assertive opens up new lines of communication. Your honesty allows the other person equal space to be honest, so the disagreement, if there is one, is brought out into the open and dealt with there.

EXERCISE 3

List those things that you do for other people because they ask you, not because you want to do them. List under work, friendship and home.

Work	Friendship	Home

Swap lists with a friend and role play, practising saying 'no' politely, for example:

> 'Can I borrow your car please?'

> 'No, Antonio, I never lend my car to anyone but family. Why don't you try hiring one?'

OTHER WAYS OF SAYING 'NO'

➤ Learn to notice your immediate 'gut response' when a request is made. Try to identify reactions, and which signal uncertainty, doubt or uneasiness. If you experience these, your answer should be 'no'.

➤ If in doubt, allow yourself to hesitate. You are not obliged to make an instant decision. Give yourself breathing space before committing yourself. Acknowledge your uncertainty and ask for qualifying information about what the commitment would entail if you agreed to the request: 'If I were to accept, what would my responsibilities be?', 'I think I would like to do it, but I need time to think. I'll get back to you by next Wednesday', 'If I said yes, would you be able to support me if X, Y, or Z happened?'

➤ If the person making the request tries to draw you into debate or asks you to change your mind, repeat your refusal calmly and clearly. Try using the 'stuck record' technique. Use the same wording exactly and they will soon respect your resolve.

➤ Take responsibility for saying 'no'. Do not blame someone else, and do not apologise.

➤ Change the conversation afterwards to avoid lingering on what may be perceived as an unpleasant topic.

➤ Identify your immediate feelings and acknowledge the difficulty honestly: 'It's difficult for me to say this, but no', or 'I feel uncomfortable saying this, but the answer is no'.

➤ Use 'I' language to show that you have a strong belief in your own judgement, convictions and decisions.

➤ Do not overuse 'fillers': 'I'm sorry', 'please', 'excuse me'. The over-apologetic person will say: 'Excuse me, I'm so sorry I interrupted you'. Compare this with the considerate response: 'I can see you're busy. Would tomorrow be a good time?'

Remember that you are refusing the request, not rejecting the person. Saying 'no' and surviving the guilt does get easier with practice!

EXERCISE 4

Stand opposite a friend. Say, 'yes' to your partner, while they reply 'no', really loudly and firmly. Or reply assertively to the questions from the following list. Swap roles. Discuss how it feels to be the recipient of a firm 'no'. Practice saying 'no' assertively, without apology or aggression.

'Would you like to stay for a cup of tea? My daughter's arriving and she'd love to meet you.'

'Can you pop this document into Chloe's house on your way home? I haven't got a car today.'

'Can you give Mr M an extra 20 minutes' treatment today, as I have a hospital appointment and I won't be back until 5 pm?'

'Can you be quick on that phone as I need to use it?'

'Do you mind if you see your clients in this room today as we are holding an exhibition in the room you usually use?'

'Can I borrow this book?'

'Can I borrow your car please – I have got visits to do and mine is right out of petrol?'

'Have you got a minute?'

'Can you take a stint on reception? M is away and they are very rushed.'

'Can you sort out the light bulb in the toilet, it's gone again?'

'Someone's been sick in the waiting room – the nurses are busy, so can you clear it up?'

'You will need to change that meeting date, as I've got to drive Poppy to her violin lesson.'

'There's no need to go to that meeting.'

MAKING REQUESTS

Learn to ask for what you want with clarity and without aggression. You have a right to make your wants known to others, remembering that they too have the right to say 'no'.

Ask for what you want specifically and directly. If you ask indirectly or drop hints, you run the risk of not being heard or being misunderstood and your request may go unheeded as a consequence. Be clear and honest. Practise asking for what you want without guise. Instead of the non-assertive, begrudging 'I suppose I ought to go and make the coffee', or 'Why is it always me that makes the coffee?', try 'Pramita, can you make the coffee today please?'. Instead of looking for support among your colleagues about how your manager does not understand the concept of working women, try: 'Can we make the meeting a little earlier to give those of us with children plenty of time to set off?' People will not know automatically or through telepathy how difficult you are finding it all unless you tell them. Learn to take charge of a situation and give yourself the permission and authority to ask for what you want.

KEY POINTS

➤ Women are taught to give up their own needs readily in order that someone else feels comfortable. They are taught, both overtly and subtly, that their own needs should come last. In delegating, we learn more about the power of equality, of real choice. We learn to be assertive and to share.

➤ It is hard to give a firm and clear 'no' when you have been socialised to be more compliant, to apologise, to have lower confidence in yourself and your abilities and rights. As a woman, one way you can regain some power, and learn to stand up for yourself and your needs, is to take a critical look at how you present as a woman.

➤ Some of the common misconceptions about saying 'no' are that saying 'no' is selfish, rude and blunt. We fear people will not like us or will take offence; we fear conflict. However, our honesty allows the other person equal space to be honest, so the disagreement, if there is one, is brought out into the open and dealt with there.

➤ How to say 'no'. If you experience uncomfortable feelings when asked, your answer should be 'no'. If in doubt, allow yourself to hesitate before committing yourself. Acknowledge any uncertainties. Use the 'stuck record' technique: repeat your refusal calmly and clearly. Take responsibility for saying 'no' – do not blame someone else and do not apologise. Do not overuse 'fillers'. Remember that you are refusing the request, not rejecting the person.

➤ When making requests, ask with clarity and without aggression. You have a right to make your wants known to others, remembering that they too have the right to say 'no'. Be specific, direct and honest; take charge and give yourself the permission and authority to ask for what you want.

CHAPTER 8

Negotiation

A negotiation may be defined as trying to reach an agreement or compromise by discussion. As this occurs many times daily in our lives, it is an important skill to get right. There are many situations when we find ourselves negotiating, either formally or informally. Informal negotiations occur whenever we are approached and asked to do something, when one party says 'no' or wishes to redefine or set limits on the activity. Formal negotiations occur on a larger scale – between governments and trade union officials, for example. This chapter identifies the skills and knowledge required to negotiate effectively.

Women are traditionally not considered to be good negotiators, as they are perceived to lack the skills of assertiveness, power, self-reliance and rationality. Some research has shown, however, that in certain circumstances, when resources are plentiful, when the woman holds a senior role, or when women negotiate on behalf of others, they are regarded as negotiating as well as men. Although we as women may choose to ignore how we are perceived during negotiations, if the outcome is not as we desire, we may have to change tactics and pander to those who are gender-sensitive. Women may need to work more to develop some of the hard-line negotiation skills, but they have an advantage with the social skills needed, if they fine-tune their well-developed interpersonal communication skills.

It is said there are two main skills used by negotiators: diagnostic and social skills. People with good diagnostic skills are able to probe and analyse, and the basic social skills are the ability to listen, question, clarify and manage the feelings involved. With this in mind, think a little about your own skill set, and how good you are at reaching mutually comfortable agreements with those you associate with. To gain some insight into your essential behaviour, it may help to use imagery – think of yourself as an animal. In negotiations, would these behaviour tendencies mark you as aggressive, passive, manipulative or assertive?

EXERCISE 1

The pigeon: you are good at your work, liked and respected by all, but do not get promoted.

The chameleon: you have become indistinguishable from the surrounding scenery – you do a good job but nobody knows it.

The wild-cat: when things do not go your way, you become aggressive – your own worst enemy.

The sloth: you have potential, but somehow never get organised in your work so your ability is never mobilised for your own advancement.

The whining watchdog: you constantly complain about work demands, the work environment, the way people behave towards you – and you are always on the lookout for something to complain of.

The willing horse: smiling sweetly, you say yes to every request.

The mule: For fear of being exploited, you object to every request.

However you currently present, you can develop negotiation skills through developing your people skills. Use good diagnostic skills: listen, really listen and keep your eyes, ears and intuition open to all the non-verbal behaviours going on in the room. Seek to understand the other person's perspective through watching, asking, analysing. These are advanced interpersonal communication skills – use them to your advantage. Question, clarify and manage the feelings involved. Develop a positive attitude, but be alert to the possibility of distractions: use your powers of observation. If you summarise often you will aid your own understanding. Prepare to feel stressed, but try to remain cool to retain your credibility.

EXERCISE 2

1   Note down five qualities that you feel describe negotiating.
2   Referring to negotiations that you have been involved in, jot down the factors that helped them to succeed.
3   What do you see as the main differences between negotiating as a team and negotiating as an individual?

A commonly held view is that negotiating means getting your own way. This may not be the case. A better definition may be *discussion producing mutual settlement or compromise*. Negotiation is not about winning at someone else's expense. It is both desirable and necessary that both parties leave the discussion feeling they have gained something. It is about managing – and avoiding

– conflict. There should be movement in both parties – concessions are made only in return for something else. In protracted or formal negotiations, both parties could shift or move their position some considerable way.

HOW TO NEGOTIATE

There are four main stages to negotiations:
1 preparation, including working out your overall aim, your strategy and objectives
2 tactics and strategies to employ during the negotiation
3 negotiating to establish an overlap, common ground
4 reaching the agreement.

1   Preparation

Before embarking on a negotiation, prepare as follows.

➤ Chose your objectives and make certain they are realistic. For example, you want a break from work – would you like an extended holiday, unpaid leave or a sabbatical? Would it be better to change from full-time to part-time working? Flexible working? Could you arrange a job share?

➤ Look at the results of previous negotiations and what others have been granted in similar positions. Is paid study leave the norm in your organisation? Has any other member of staff had their hours changed favourably?

➤ Assess your own negotiating power. Look realistically at what you are worth in your job. What is your commitment to the organisation? What does your track record look like?

➤ Understand, the other party's plan and position. What is their position in the hierarchy? What specific limitations are to be expected? How far are they able to grant you your request, or will they need to seek higher authority?

➤ Be aware of the personal and political constraints held by the other party. What will they gain from your plan? Be aware of some of the arguments they are likely to use and prepare your response.

Both parties need to understand the negotiating procedures and the jargon used.

➤ What is your 'fall back' position (the least you are prepared to settle for)?

➤ What 'concessions' are you willing to make (those things you are prepared to give up to gain what you want)?

➤ What are the consequences of withdrawal? You can refuse to continue negotiations if they become unfavourable, but plan a strategic withdrawal rather than just walking out – this may cause you to lose face if the talks are resumed at a later date.

➤ What is the 'hidden agenda'? Be aware of the undercurrents.

➤ Prepare a contingency plan if you fail to achieve what you want.

➤ Choose the right time and place. Avoid a time when the opposition may be under pressure, and clarify with them beforehand what you want to discuss so that they also have time to prepare.

When preparing to negotiate, be clear about your outcome and work out the strategies to be used beforehand: role play or note them down. Avoid using a straight 'no'. There is a need to establish some sort of overlap with the other party because without common ground and understanding, negotiation becomes impossible. Be prepared to move your ground, even if only slightly. You will need to frame and develop a positive attitude and be aware of distractions used or side issues and irrelevancies thrown up by the other party that may confuse the issue. If this happens, be firm and ask for clarification, or reaffirm the issue in hand: use your powers of observation and summarise frequently to aid understanding.

2 Tactics during the negotiation

➤ Try not to use threatening or provocative behaviours.

➤ If you make a threat at any stage, you need to be prepared to follow it through.

➤ Find common ground – you want both parties to leave the negotiation feeling successful.

➤ Test, understand and summarise.

➤ Evaluate.

➤ If in doubt, be prepared to adjourn.

Avoid

➤ Words with emotive content: 'A generous offer', for example.

➤ Spirals of defend and attack.

➤ Counter proposals.

➤ Position taking.

Successful negotiators explore a wide bargaining range and plot issues separately, breaking items down into smaller units for discussion. Clarification and questioning skills are essential skills in this procedure. Assertive skills that need to be used are the 'stuck record' technique: the need to repeat oneself if the other party goes off at a tangent, has misunderstood or is using distracting side issues. You need to be able to empathise with the other party, and acknowledge you have understood their position: 'I can see that you are unhappy about it, but I cannot complete the work today. I could finish it by Tuesday though' – state your compromise.

There can be a lot of stress involved in some confrontations, and emotions and feelings run high. Try to remain cool. Retain your credibility. Be aware of, and be proud of, your own skills. Use your knowledge of these in the bargaining procedure.

Be clear and specific
➤ Make the statement simple, brief and direct.
➤ Own your statement, assume responsibility.
➤ Be firm and clear, avoid unnecessary padding.
➤ Seek clarity from the other party if you are not sure, or feel muddled and unhappy.
➤ Clarity untangles unexpressed needs or manipulation.
➤ When you express a willingness to accept the situation and look at changing it, you regain the power.

Be open and honest about your feelings
➤ Take personal responsibility for your feelings.
➤ Begin difficult situations with simple statements, for example: 'I feel nervous … I know this is difficult for both of us …' The immediate effect is to defuse or reduce your anxiety, enabling you to relax and take charge of yourself and your feelings.
➤ Self-disclosure demonstrates that you have a greater acceptance of all the aspects of your personality, which shows greater maturity and professionalism.

Repeat your message
➤ Remember the 'stuck record' technique: if you feel misheard, calmly repeat your statement or request.
➤ Maintain your position without being influenced by manipulative comment, irrelevant logic or argumentative bait: the negotiators will accept and respect your clarity, determination and ability to set your own priorities.

Listen, understand, but do not necessarily agree
➤ Listen carefully to the other person's point of view, acknowledge it and then stick to your desired point.
➤ Do not be led by anyone else's aim to control the agenda. This is your agenda, so avoid any diversion by clever and articulate argument. Stay with what you need, relax and keep to your word.
➤ Indicate that you have heard what is said; acknowledge the other person's point of view, while still continuing confidently with your request or statement.

Demonstrate you are able to understand the other person's point of view, even though you do not necessarily share it. If attempts are made to undermine you with criticism, 'read' behind the statement, and either acknowledge it as fair or dismiss it as irrelevant. Remember and employ the techniques learnt in the previous chapter, in making and refusing requests.

➤ Prompt others to express themselves.
➤ Seek out criticism about yourself.
➤ Prompt negative feelings.

When behaving assertively, you are confronting issues and situations rather than waiting passively in the hope that you will be able to respond. It is less stressful, and more powerful, to set the agenda yourself. As you take charge of the agenda, you communicate more powerfully. You then take the risk of opening the levels of communication. Thus, you must expect honest communication back, probably including some criticism of parts of your work. Accept constructive criticism if it is fair or truthful: acknowledge the truth, take up the opportunities offered to change the situation around positively – offer positive alternatives. In this way you demonstrate that you remain your own judge.

As a woman, if you are negotiating with a team that is gender-sensitive and finding it hard to take you seriously, you may need to behave slightly differently, due to the preconceptions of your colleagues. Build up your ability, experience and work role, arguing from your position rather than your personality, and reinforce the idea that you are negotiating on behalf of your team or department, not yourself.[1]

➤ Frame your request in terms of your contribution to the department. This reinforces your concern for others, your caring side, and that you espouse community.
➤ Appeal to common goals across departments, stressing co-operation.
➤ If you are negotiating in the role of team leader, remind your negotiators that you are negotiating on behalf of all members.
➤ Stress any 'out of norm' behaviour: 'normally, this issue would not bother me, but …'

3   The negotiation

➤ Plan for strategic withdrawal if you need time to think: adjourn.
➤ What is the 'hidden agenda'? Be aware of the undercurrents.
➤ Remember it will be unusual if you get your own way entirely.
➤ You will have a discussion, hopefully producing mutual settlement or compromise.

---

1 Tinsley CH, Cheldelin S, Schneider AK, *et al*. Women at the bargaining table: pitfalls and prospects. *Negotiation Journal*. 2009; **25**(2): 233.

➤ There should be movement in both parties – concessions are made only in return for something else.

➤ Remember that both parties could shift or move their position some considerable way.

➤ Both parties need to leave the discussion feeling they have gained something.

➤ Avoid personal argument.

➤ Negotiate from an equal position.

➤ Be proud of your own skills.

➤ State your compromise, but never compromise on your self-respect.

4   Having reached an agreement

➤ Guidelines should be established regarding any agreements reached.

➤ Check for follow-up.

➤ Check dates specified for implementation.

Both parties should leave the negotiating table feeling happy about the outcome. Guidelines should be established regarding any agreements reached, any follow-up required and dates specified for implementation.

EXAMPLE 3

Here we use an example of a practice manager, employed in general practice, using a range of successful tactics in negotiating a pay rise.

Preparation

Do your homework first: familiarise yourself with both the grades and rates of pay, getting copies of relevant pay scales as guide lines, with outline job descriptions to match suggested grades. Check to see if you feel you are being paid unfairly, and see whether there are any areas of work that you currently undertake that are not reflected in your current rate of pay, and any areas you aspire to that you could offer as added value to the organisation.

Always ask for more pay if you take on any job that is clearly more substantial in terms of responsibility: for example, if you are now taking responsibility for a block of work single-handedly whereas before you worked under supervision. Use the scales and grades as a guideline to support your case. Before even considering embarking on a negotiation, chose your objectives and make certain they are realistic.

The practice manager's agenda

Look at the results of previous negotiations and what others have been granted in similar positions.

➤ What is the general rate of pay for managers with a practice your size in your area?
➤ Look honestly at what you are worth in your job.
➤ Look honestly at the pay scales.
➤ What is your commitment to the organisation?
➤ What does your track record look like?
➤ What 'extras' can you offer?
➤ What is your fall-back position (the least you are prepared to settle for)?
➤ What concessions are you willing to make? More hours for more pay? Reduced holiday?
➤ Prepare a contingency plan. For example, an ideal settlement might be a 5% increase, a realistic settlement 3% and the fall-back position increased holiday.
➤ What would it feel like to lose? Be prepared for this.

The GP's agenda

Be aware of some of the arguments that are likely to be used and prepare your response.
➤ Look at, and understand, the GP's plan: they will not want to pay any more, but they might want to keep you: it may be an awkward time for you to leave – capitalise on this.
➤ Do they want you to further your role?
➤ What will they gain from your plan?
➤ Can they afford you?
➤ Will they be able to support your claim to the commissioners/health authority/funders if they want to increase any amount they are being reimbursed or subsidised?
➤ What are their present profit levels like? Are they bemoaning the fact they have not had a pay rise in the last three years – if so, it is not a good time for you to act. Wait until they are more buoyant, or until you have brought a large sum of money into the practice or received outside accolades.

Fall back position: if they do not want to pay you, go for enhanced non-pay items: increased holiday, enhanced benefits. Be prepared for the partners to refuse point blank, but it is more likely they will redefine your terms or set limits: remember to concede some things; they need to feel they have gained something too from the discussions.

Before the negotiation

➤ Choose the right time and place, clear time and space for your needs to be heard, avoiding a time when the 'opposition' may be under pressure.
➤ Clarify with them beforehand what you want to discuss so that they also have time to prepare.

➤ Write a letter outlining your case, and ask to meet the partners to discuss the matter.

➤ This is a formal negotiation: do not let it be by-passed or undermined as a side issue in another, impromptu meeting.

➤ If necessary, rehearse with sympathetic friends or colleagues.

➤ Speak positively about *when* you take on your new role, not *if*.

Listen, understand, but do not necessarily agree

When you are negotiating with someone in a position of authority, such as your employer, take care not to be led by their aim to control the agenda. This is your agenda, so avoid any diversion by clever and articulate argument. Stay with what you need, relax and keep to your word. You can indicate that you have heard what is said and acknowledge the other person's point of view, while still continuing confidently with your request or statement.

> 'I understand that you are concerned about your own drop in pay over the last year or so, and this is something I am sure you have taken up with the appropriate authorities. My concern is with my pay and conditions of work, and this is what we need to get back to now.'

There may be attempts to undermine you with criticism: 'But you are never available now when I want to see you, if you did this new work we would never see you.' If this is so, remember the techniques you have learned about accepting or fending off criticism. Is this fair or unfair? Are you being manipulated?

The above request hides frustration and resentment. 'Read' behind the statement, so that your response could begin:

> 'Yes, I am often away from the office when you need me. Unfortunately this job does necessitate me being away in meetings fairly frequently, and this will increase as I increase my responsibilities outside the practice. What we need to think about is how I can best meet the practice need to stay in touch – how about more one to one meetings/using my mobile to keep in touch?'

State your compromise.

To retain your position of power and your own authority, use the assertive skill of prompting others to express themselves. In this context, it exposes the criticism and encourages your critics to be more assertive. For example, you may ask: 'Are you finding this difficult to talk about – money always is!' or 'Do you think I'm being unfair?'. In behaving assertively, you are confronting issues and situations rather than waiting passively. Set the agenda yourself, take charge. You do run the risk of honest communication back, probably including some criticism of parts of your work, but now is the time to understand yourself and accept constructive criticism if it is fair or truthful.

Examples of your response may be 'Yes, I know I can be aggressive at times' and 'You are right. People management is not my best skill. However, we could take this opportunity to build on my strengths and minimise my weaknesses. If I delegate all first line management to X, who is brilliant at it, that would free me up to concentrate on policy and planning'.

In acknowledging the truth, you demonstrate that you remain your own judge, and now is the time to take up the opportunities offered to change the situation around positively: open up the discussions to offer a range of positive alternatives.

SUMMARY OF THE STAGES IN THE NEGOTIATING PROCESS

➤ Work out a strategy, remembering timing is very important.
➤ Decide on objectives: for example, 'I want an 8% pay increase', 'I would like a three-week holiday in June'.
➤ Assess your own and others' negotiating power: for example, 'What am I worth in my job?', 'What is my commitment to the organisation?', 'My past experience?, 'What is my boss's position in the hierarchy?'.
➤ Establish specific objectives:
  – the ideal settlement: 8% increase in pay?
  – a realistic settlement: 5% increase in pay?
  – the fall-back position: 4% increase in pay?
➤ Establish overlap with the other party.

Remember that there can be a lot of stress involved in some confrontation situations and emotions can run high. Build up your credibility and respond to the others' expectations.

EMPOWERMENT AND INNOVATION

Being assertive is a very powerful and freeing tool. When we behave assertively, we experience positive feelings, which reinforce our own strength and stability, and allow us to have more influence and authority in life. In learning to be assertive, you are releasing untapped potential and beginning a process of self-discovery through which you can begin really to understand yourself, and others, more. Through being assertive you also empower others, allowing them the room to take space and negotiate their needs. As your sensitivity to others increases, so will your ability to negotiate well, as will your ability to understand the other parties' perspective and feel care and compassion for them too.

KEY POINTS

➤ A commonly held view is that negotiating means getting your own way. This may not be the case. A better definition may be *discussion producing mutual settlement or compromise.* Negotiation is not about winning at someone else's expense.

➤ Women may need to work harder to develop some of the hard-line negotiation skills, but they have an advantage with their fine-tuned interpersonal communication skills.

➤ It is said there are two main skills used by negotiators: diagnostic and social skills. People with good diagnostic skills are able to probe and analyse; while the basic social skills are the ability to listen, question, clarify and manage the feelings involved.

➤ There are four main stages to negotiations:
  1 preparation, including working out your overall aim, objectives, concessions, and strategy
  2 tactics and strategies to employ during the negotiation
  3 negotiating to establish an overlap, common ground
  4 reaching the agreement.

➤ Understand the other side's constraints and clarify what they will gain. There is a need to establish some sort of overlap with the other party, because without common ground and understanding, negotiation becomes impossible.

➤ Avoid words with emotive content, spirals of defend and attack, counter-proposals, and position taking.

➤ Successful negotiators explore their bargaining range and plot issues separately, break items down into smaller units for discussion, use clarification and questioning skills, and remain cool.

➤ Baseline negotiation skills are to: be clear and specific, open and honest; repeat your message; listen; understand, but not necessarily agree; and use assertive criticism techniques.

➤ Both parties should leave the negotiating table feeling happy about the outcome. Guidelines should be established regarding any agreements reached, any follow up required and dates specified for implementation.

➤ By being assertive, you also empower others, allowing them the room to take space and negotiate their needs. As your sensitivity to others increases, so will your ability to negotiate well, as will your ability to understand the other parties' perspective.

CHAPTER 9

Preventing and resolving conflict

Conflict resolution is not about breakaway techniques but about models of communication, and how to de-escalate, diffuse or resolve conflict.

This chapter looks more closely at some of the useful skills to adopt that will assist in preventing and resolving conflicts, both personal and at work. We look at what anger is, how we can learn to manage it, some common work situations where conflict arises and some strategies for managing these difficulties.

In all work situations, there will be conflicts that should be avoided and conflicts that should be managed. In the long term, it is harder to feel conflicted when we understand ourselves fully, are open and honest with ourselves and others, and recognise and accept differences between individuals and groups, in terms of values, perceptions, expectations and needs.[1] Section 4 examines some of these differences in more detail: if you feel you need more insight into why conflict occurs, I refer you to this section next. It is possible to prevent conflicts from arising if we allocate sufficient time and energy to really get to know the people we work with, so that we understand their values, beliefs, etc. Never automatically assume that you are right and they are wrong, and be alert to your own feelings of defensiveness if others disagree with your ideas. If we provide suitable ways in which people can express their feelings about things, we ensure that we learn from previous conflicts that have been resolved, and living is more harmonious.

The main causes of conflict occur through:

➤ expectations not being met
➤ lack of information
➤ poor communication
➤ inconvenience to the consumer, for example, long waiting times, cancelled appointments
➤ poor attitudes.

---

1 Pryor F. Conference papers. Fred Pryor Seminars; 1994. Available at: www.pryor.com (accessed April 2013).

Conflict occurs where there are opposed principles, incompatibility: when we do not share the same values. Patterns of conflict range from compliance and verbal resistance through to aggressive or serious/aggravated resistance. The good news is that as you develop your assertiveness skills, you will find it easier to let go of your anger, as well as to manage conflict from others. In this chapter, we look at some suggestions on managing both.

ANGER

Anger is a very early, basic emotion. It is said by psychologists to be released through our fears; our search for security, belonging and conformity; our tribalism and submissiveness to leaders.[2] If our defences are threatened, we have a reliable self-protection system that picks up on the threat and gives us a burst of feelings such as anger, anxiety or disgust. These feelings ripple through our bodies, alerting us and urging us to take action against the threat – to protect ourselves. They can be painful and difficult; they may cajole us into an instant response or inhibit us so we freeze or submit.

Inappropriate and often violent expressions of anger and aggression are on the increase in our society, and we need to employ techniques both effectively to control our own anger and to cope with other people. Here are some statements that have been made about anger.

➤ Anger affects our bodies, health and minds.
➤ It is physically impossible to be relaxed and angry at the same time.
➤ There is a connection between anger, underlying hurt and depression.
➤ We cannot think clearly when we are gripped by the force of any emotion – especially anger.
➤ Venting the anger does not make it go away – it can make it worse.
➤ Uncontrolled anger is an emotionally driven trance state.
➤ It is possible to learn to see things from a different perspective.
➤ It is possible to inoculate yourself against stress build up.
➤ Anger – and the build up of cortisol, the stress hormone – can have a devastating impact on your immune system and long-term health.

An uncontrolled/aggressive reaction is most common in all of us when we feel under threat, usually as a result of criticism. We react instantly: we rise to the bait easily and use defensive behaviour to deflect the comment in our defence. This sort of reaction is never constructive, and can lead quickly to heated argument. This is not an appropriate way to behave in a work situation,

---

2   Gilbert P. *The Compassionate Mind: a new approach to life's challenges.* Kindle ed. Constable; 2010. pp. 336, 472.

but it can and does occur. If you find things have developed in this way, there is a need for apology on both sides: one to acknowledge the provocation and one for reacting in such an uncontrollable way.

Anger is engendered by our expectation of unacceptable behaviour on the part of others. Our attitudes and behaviour are shaped by our experiences, beliefs, our own needs and values, socio-economic variances, and the attitudes of others towards us.

Thus, there will always be a mismatch between what each of us considers acceptable behaviour. The aim is to try to understand each other's world, and find common ground. What do we know and assume about anger? First, check out your automatic behaviours, assumptions, prejudices, value systems and trust of others with the following questions.

EXERCISE 1

➤ What do people most frequently consult with in healthcare systems? Mental health problems? Problems related to long-term, chronic disabilities? Why is it that we are often reluctant to provide a service for these groups of people, given that they make up the work we choose to do?

➤ What would it take for you to leave your family, friends and culture and go to live in a place where you knew nobody, did not speak the language and were not permitted to work? What qualities do you think you would need to do so? Stamina? Drive? Bravery? Do we equip asylum seekers with these qualities? Why not?

➤ When you notice people in shopping malls, do you think some of them are unemployed, just wandering around since they have nothing better to do? Or are they just shopping, exercising or visiting with friends, like you?

➤ How impatient and ready to anger are you? When a person with you speaks slowly, do you listen until the person finishes talking? Or do you cut them off and finish off their statement? When you are a front seat passenger, do you stay alert and watchful or relax and enjoy the view? While your partner is cooking dinner, do you keep them company, chat about your day while waiting, or occasionally check in on them to see what they are doing and make sure the food does not overcook?

➤ When you notice someone in a restaurant who is obese, do you acknowledge that she may have physical or psychological difficulties, or wonder secretly why she cannot control her food intake?

Reasons for anger

Dealing with other's unwanted emotions is stressful. Oliver James notes that self-hatred, the root of some of the out-of-control behaviour we see in patients/

clients, can turn towards others.[3] Many healthcare workers become dustbins for their client's anger and self-hatred. Clients may unconsciously project these unwanted feelings, in a covert or overt way: by missing appointments, keeping professionals waiting for appointments or making veiled suicide threats. Flows of aggression and depression can run in families – we pass or dump from one to another, and get rid of our own angry, critical feelings by inducing them in another, thus moving from an 'I'm not ok, you are ok' position to 'I'm ok, you're not'. Self-hatred raises the thought that killers stab or smash feelings held inside themselves, and rapists ejaculate their 'badness' into their victims. Those who commit or attempt suicide plague their loved ones with guilt, depression and rage: 'Look what you've made me do.' Both those who kill and those who kill themselves are thus paralysed by self-loathing. James cites that three-quarters of convicted violent men are depressed, and become more depressed and aggressive when locked up. Depression can make those with aggressive tendencies violent to their partners and others. There is a fluidity of depression/aggression, where the pain is felt, then passed back.

How do we respond to anger?

We can be frightened of anger, especially when our patients or clients behave aggressively, and this fear can cause us to react in one of many defensive ways.

➤ We ignore: speak in a light, bright and cheerful voice which avoids acknowledgement of the pain and forces the listener to push down and suppress the distress quickly.

➤ We placate and comply: we avoid eye contact, give a too-pleasant smile, and agree with the patient or give way to their demands.

➤ We are over-knowledgeable – we try to blind people with science, using long words and explanations, insisting that if they do as we say everything will be all right.

➤ We control – keeping people at bay with distance and rank, quoting rules and regulations, insisting on specific behaviour or controlling the time allocation strictly.

➤ We respond angrily – we react to their distress with loudness and strong gestures, bring in staff reinforcements and accuse the patient/client of being a trouble-maker.

If any of the above are common patterns of response for you, check the motives behind your behaviour. Some danger signs are your own hurt, envy, resentment, resistance or desire to retaliate. Are you operating according to your principles or in response to theirs? Think about your intention in the interaction. Is it to manipulate, hurt, teach a lesson or resolve the issue?

---

3 James O. Dealing with aggression. *Community Care*. 1999 Mar 12. pp. 4–10.

To help you to understand your own responses a little more, look for recurring patterns in your life.

➤ Who makes you angry?
➤ What events trigger your anger? Someone not listening to you? (Challenge this – take charge: 'It's important for me to be heard here. My feelings do count.')
➤ When and with whom do you feel safe enough to express your anger?
➤ What are the messages you have heard about anger?
➤ What happens to your body when you feel angry?
➤ What physical ways do you have for letting of steam?

WAYS TO MANAGE YOUR OWN ANGER

As you develop your assertion skills, you will find that you are more inclined to rid yourself of anger. There are some common obstacles to getting rid of this anger. If you try to adopt some of the healthier approaches outlined in this chapter, possibly using the behavioural experiment sheets or another cognitive behaviour therapy approach,[4] you will go a long way towards leading a calmer, more compassionate and healthy life.

Common obstacles to managing anger[5]

Your anger is self-righteous

If you feel that your anger is justified, check that you are not falling into the self-righteous trap, not seeing that the other person is wrong and you are right: rarely is any confrontation that cut and dried; each party has to take some responsibility. If you cling to a belief that you are right, this could lead to a desire for vengeance, a desire to prove yourself through shoring up your own ego. Even if you are aware that your anger responses cause you difficulty in life, you may still find it hard to let go of them, especially if you feel you are responding through 'righteous' anger: your anger may support and justify a strong political belief, for example; you may be fighting oppression or fear being undermined. Sometimes it is hard in this context to see an alternative.[6] If it is a political belief you are holding, it may be easier at least to acknowledge a difference of opinion, and release your hold on the anger this way. However, if the conflict is less entrenched, and you allow yourself to be wrong and admit it,

---

4 Deffenbacher JL, Dahlen ER, Lynch RS, *et al.* An application of Beck's cognitive therapy to general anger reduction. *Cognitive Therapy and Research.* 2000; **24**(6): 689–97.
5 Willson R, Branch R. *Cognitive Behaviour Therapy for Dummies.* John Wiley & Sons; 2006. pp. 187–8.
6 Gilbert, note 2 above, pp. 87–8.

it is a sign of strength not one of weakness or inferiority. By admitting you are wrong, this, paradoxically, can help you feel more, not less, powerful.

Power

If you have low self-esteem, your anger may make you feel strong and powerful. You may get an adrenaline rush, you may feel invigorated and passionate. Here though, the unhealthy anger may mean you are stepping on another person's rights to express themselves: you intimidate to boost your own feelings of inadequacy. Look for other ways to boost your sense of self without undermining those around you.

Lack of empathy

Consider whether you may be unaware that you lack empathy, and are not seeing the impact of your anger on those near to you. If so, ask those around you how they feel about your anger (inviting constructive criticism). Think about the times you have been on the receiving end of unhealthy – aggressive or intimidating – behaviour and how you have felt and use this feedback to help you to change how you express your feelings in the future.

Weakness

If you feel that being angry is a sign of your strength, recall that people who are assertive gain much more respect through being firm and fair.

Anger as control

Sometimes people use anger to control others and, if so, the aggression can lead to those around them avoiding the intimidating, bullying behaviour. Do not mistake this fear for respect: it is not. People around you may comply through fear, especially if you hold any position of authority, but there is no genuine, healthy regard for you. Is this really how you want to be seen? If we routinely appeal to a higher authority, we use that authority to threaten, cajole, reward, control or punish someone else because we know our own authority and ability to persuade is not enough. So perhaps focus on other ways, using pro-social behaviour to help become kinder, compassionate and more empathic.[7]

Help avoid your own anger by building successful relationships

➤ Try to adopt a more relaxed and positive approach to people – greet them regularly by name; take time to develop social relationships with colleagues.

---

7 Mikulincer M, Shaver PR. *Attachment in Adulthood: structure, dynamics and change.* The Guilford Press; 2007. Gilbert, note 2 above, p. 82.

➤ Be more appreciative and positive in your relationships.

➤ Build understanding and respect into your relationships. Avoid demeaning: 'You've got to be kidding!', 'I thought at least you would know better'. Give yourself time to think more thoroughly and fairly about what you're going to say.

➤ Do not blame others for failing to meet your own ideals. Point out that we should all learn from our mistakes. Do not make faults in others an excuse for your own failures and disappointments.

➤ Avoid negativity: do you greet every new suggestion or request with a reason why it will not work or cannot be done? Next time someone asks you to do something, respond with a positive or alternative suggestion.

➤ Be assertive: if somebody incenses you by asking for a long document to be read and commented on at 5 pm on Friday, respond reasonably: 'I can do it tomorrow first thing, at the moment this other job takes priority', or 'I realise your job is important, but I am leaving the office now so I'll do it first thing on Monday'.

➤ Make yourself aware of the effect of your behaviour on other people, and if you think your behaviour is hostile, ask for feedback – and be prepared for frankness!

➤ Be proactive not reactive.

➤ Describe instead of interpreting.

Generally, a respect for life, people and other approaches goes a long way. As always, focus on commonalities rather than differences, and avoid gender/race/sexuality biased attitudes, categorising and generalising.

RESOLVING CONFLICTS AT WORK

It is not always possible to prevent a conflict occurring, and when one does occur, it may become necessary at least to try to resolve it in as positive and constructive a manner as possible. Successful conflict resolution has to be based on an accurate and thorough understanding of the actual conflict itself. There are five broad approaches to successful conflict resolution. The approach adopted should match the particular characteristics and circumstances of the conflict situation. Although some of the approaches may appear less than assertive and honest, there is room for considering a more tactful, conciliatory approach if the context is complex or the situation – such as an argument between colleagues – requires adroitness and sensitivity rather than a more honest, robust approach.

➤ **Denial:** trying to solve the conflict by withdrawing, denying its existence. This can be satisfactory if the conflict is relatively unimportant, or if there is a need for a cooling-off period before the conflict is tackled head on.

➤ **Suppression:** differences are played down, and a harmonious facade is constructed. Again, this approach can be satisfactory for relatively unimportant conflicts, or for situations where the relationship between the two parties in conflict must be preserved at all costs.

➤ **Domination:** the conflict is resolved by one party using their authority or position. This approach can be satisfactory where the domination is based on clear authority or where the approach has been agreed on by the parties involved.

➤ **Compromise:** resolution occurs when each party gives something up in order to meet half way. This approach can be satisfactory if both parties have sufficient room to alter their positions, although overall commitment to the 'agreed upon' solution may be in doubt.

➤ **Collaboration:** individual differences are recognised, and the aim is for group consensus, so all participants feel that they have won. This approach can be satisfactory if there is the time available and the individuals believe in the approach and have the necessary skills.

Conflicts are part of normal everyday life: too few, and life is boring; too many and life can become stressful. Conflicts are nearly always caused by people having different points of view, or by people trying to achieve what they want at the expense of others. Some of the principal causes of conflict at work are:

➤ misunderstandings
➤ personality clashes
➤ differences in goals/methods to be used
➤ substandard performance
➤ problems relating to areas of responsibility and authority
➤ lack of co-operation
➤ frustration
➤ competition for limited resources
➤ non-compliance with rules and policies.

Managers spend much of their time at work dealing with conflict. However, there are positive and negative aspects of conflict in organisations. Conflict can be positive when it helps to open up discussion of an issue or results in problems being solved. Then it can increase the level of individual involvement and interest in an issue, improve communication between people and even safely release emotions that have been stored up. The resolution of conflict then helps people to develop their interpersonal communication and work skills and abilities.

However, we are all aware that conflict can be negative when it diverts people from dealing with the really important issues, creates feelings of dissatisfaction among the people involved and leads to individuals and groups becoming insular and unco-operative.

Conflicts that are likely to result in positive outcomes are to be encouraged in organisations. And negative-outcome conflicts should be either prevented or resolved in a positive manner. Over the years, most managers will have developed a number of approaches to such situations, based on their own experiences. The effective manager is one who is able to draw on a wide range of approaches, and is able to apply them to situations that are fully understood. Understanding the nature and causes of conflict at work, and being able to use a wide range of approaches to prevent and resolve conflict, are essential for anyone with managerial responsibilities.

Dealing with complaints from the public

The best way of dealing with complaints and provocative or aggressive behaviour is to be proactive, so you both minimise the complaints and prepare ahead for their resolution. The maxim is to:

➤ keep people informed
➤ provide the very best service you can afford
➤ respect the expectation for clean, tidy, private and well-kept premises
➤ display any relevant policies and procedures, such as for complaints or repeat prescriptions, and supply a system for keeping people informed about delays
➤ make certain records are available when the patient/client consults
➤ audit complaints and plaudits, categorise the reason for the failure, be open about naming the person responsible, collectively discuss ways to solve the problem, and implement them
➤ give people copies of correspondence relating to them, with a glossary of medical abbreviations and terms
➤ train all staff to be welcoming, attentive, helpful, and to keep negative opinions to themselves.

Within caring services, common negative experiences are usually due to lack of information, poor communication, with either the public or other professionals or within the system. Complaints also commonly arise when there are obvious variations in provisions, bureaucracy and hierarchies that are perceived to be benefiting the system not the patient/client, and a lack of understanding/acknowledgement of the real, emotional issues affecting the client and carers.

Any good initiative has at its root good, or better, communication between patient, professionals and staff. Consider some of the more recent NHS initiatives and note who benefits most, and why.

National service frameworks.
Local centres of excellence.
Collaborative care planning.
Patient forums.
Primary/secondary care protocols.
More screening.
Carer groups.
Individual and local initiatives, for example, taped consultations in cancer care.
Expert patient forums.

Despite our best efforts, many people do experience problems within the system, and complain. When this happens, the role of the manager is not to ignore, but to pull together the evidence and present it back to his or her team so it can inform future, better practice.

According to a millennium report from the General Medical Services,[8] the most common complaints needing resolution from general practice concern poor communication, inappropriate or ineffective care management, or the complainer having some association with grief, or delayed or failed diagnosis.

Some solutions

It is crucial to apologise immediately if you are in the wrong. An apology given over the phone results in a higher level of complaints being resolved than an apology by letter. Put the problem right immediately – do not cause those complaining further delay or anguish. Your response must be real and important to you, otherwise it will be perceived as a standard, and impersonal, business response:

➤ apologise first, explaining who responsible without apportioning specific blame
➤ acknowledge the complainer's anxiety using clear language
➤ acknowledge and understand the problem you have caused them
➤ then give an explanation, but only if it is essential
➤ finish with how you are going to put it right
➤ thank the complainer for drawing your attention to the matter.

---

8   Green DR. The rising tide of complaints. *Pulse*. 2000 Dec 15.

EXAMPLE

A patient telephones her local GP practice to change a date with the practice counsellor. The message is relayed wrongly, and the patient subsequently arrives expecting to see the counsellor, who is absent on that day. The subsequent apology, by phone or letter, should include some of the following text:

> 'I do apologise on behalf of the practice for the mix-up regarding your cancellation, which meant that we did not get to meet today. It must have been very difficult to arrive and find I was not there. Unfortunately, I understood the cancellation referred to X date. I am so sorry that our work was unexpectedly disrupted. The practice will of course give you a further session. I look forward to seeing you again on Y.'

HOW TO HANDLE DIFFICULT PEOPLE OR SITUATIONS

How do you react when you are worried and panicky? It may be that you can remain reasonable and considerate most of the time, but break under certain situations: if someone cries, or is angry, or it is the fourth complaint that day.

➤ If your client is *frightened*, they need you to take charge. Move them to a private space, acknowledge their distress, and handle the situation with sympathy, competence and firm reassurance.

➤ If your client not fully *competent*, they need you to take charge: clarify essential details such as name, phone number, address; provide accessible, compassionate and kindly help; and avoid spelling out the rules.

➤ If the patient is *deeply distressed* and you have the unhappy task of communicating unwelcome news, try these ideas. It is said that bad news is to be shared, not broken, as what is broken cannot be mended.[9]

➤ Think about body language, eye contact and language use.

➤ Never use euphemisms – they are unclear communication and misunderstandings will happen.

➤ Be clear, direct and honest.

➤ Look people in the eye.

➤ Sit next to or close to the person.

➤ If necessary, back up the news by reading any related correspondence together – people forget when distressed, and remembering seeing it written down reinforces it.

➤ Tape important conversations.

---

9 Jennings T. Clinical casebook: preparing the ground for breaking bad news. *Registrar Pulse.* 2001 Jun 30. p. 47.

➤ Communicate honestly and without defence: clients and relatives have a right to know.
➤ Keep checking that you have been understood.
➤ Make use of trained staff – psychologists and counsellors to supervise and debrief, not doctors.
➤ Do not use humour and flippancy to defend yourself against the feelings – you are not the one that needs the defences.
➤ If the client is *defensive*, avoid the triggers for defensive behaviour: which are control, blame, judgement, indifference and misinformation.
➤ If the patient is *crying and out of control*, wait, do not offer verbal sympathy or intervene as this might escalate the situation; use the time to collect your thoughts, while using obvious sympathetic body language: head tilt, good eye contact.
➤ If the client is *chronic complainer*:
    – ask for co-operation
    – use positive language: 'If we don't co-operate there will be problem'; 'Is there anything I can say or do that would gain your co-operation?'
    – plan ahead: 'So what do you want to see happen?'
    – take control: 'I know what you have to say is important, but I can't listen at the moment. Can we take the issue to the next staff meeting and try and solve it there?'; 'I want to make sure I understand you – let's meet tomorrow when I have more time'
    – try being silent, stop giving feedback.[10]

If you are faced with a difficult patient/client, the following tips may help.
➤ Make sure that the most appropriate member of staff is dealing with the situation: the one who feels least threatened, not the most senior necessarily.
➤ Match the emotion rather than contradicting it – if people are angry, use a strong voice; if scared, drop your voice.
➤ If extreme violence threatens, never leave it too late to call for help – make sure one member of staff on each shift has the responsibility for calling the police the minute trouble starts – otherwise everyone will think this is someone else's job.
➤ If in doubt, leave the room taking the other members of the public and staff with you. Equipment can be replaced – people cannot.

People who behave reactively are out of control; they are responding to external influences. These reactive responses are related to insecurity, unmet needs and fear, so these feelings can be negated by asking: 'How secure do you feel here?',

---

10 Pryor, note 1 above.

'Are you getting what you need from us?', or 'What are you scared of?'. Aim instead to choose a response that involves you responding, not reacting. Look for a win-win outcome.

If we have a good self-image, and self-esteem, we are able to think kindly of ourselves: 'I am someone who is thoughtful, caring, who has integrity.' Not everyone is able to do this. Good self-esteem helps us to behave assertively in difficult situations: we respect the needs of others and ourselves; we care enough to have the courage to connect – if we have awareness of, and commitment to, what we are doing. We have enough of ourselves to behave with humility. If focussed on ego, we behave arrogantly, greedily, competitively and in a self-focussed way. Perceptions that precipitate anger are self-imposed messages such as 'No one likes me', 'I must be perfect', 'Everyone must follow my rules', 'I am always right'.

Conflict will always occur when there is miscommunication, conflict between personality types, differing values, perceptions and opposing objectives. Stress occurs when our perception colours an event that has triggered us emotionally. We are more likely to react angrily if stressed. In both instances, we need to find the common ground.

STRATEGIES TO REDUCE ANGER

When someone confronts us angrily we need calmly to acknowledge the situation, and then state our feelings before discussing the priorities and alternatives. If necessary, use the 'stuck record' technique, and avoid using aggressive, non-verbal leakage such as strutting about, pointing or raising your voice. Reflective body language works in counselling, but not when faced with aggression.

Good practice indicates[11] that when shocked, we breathe rapidly: so relax, breathe deeply to signal non-aggression. Use open, free-flowing hand movements, one at a time. Avoid (and read) hand-to-head signals as these show signs of anxiety, loss of patience . They can have sexual connotations. Watch your own body language: do not fold arms to form a barrier, stand or sit at slight angle, and use good personal space. Do not touch unless serious assault is indicated: poking and pushing will escalate violence. Keep your face in tune: if you smile inappropriately it will be read as a smirk. Do establish eye contact, but remember that some cultures do not establish eye contact with people they regard as superior, so be aware of gender, culture and ethnicity differences. Discuss differences openly to learn more, interpret correctly and react appropriately.

---

11 Braithwaite R. Anger management. *Community Care*. 1999 Sep. pp. 16–22.

Avoiding conflict escalation
➤ Listen.
➤ Remain calm and centred, detached from the personality.
➤ Focus on the facts rather than the position.
➤ Create and maintain a positive atmosphere.
➤ Consider 'time out'.
➤ Identify the needs and benefits of resolution.
➤ Agree where disagreements can coexist.
➤ Look for common ground.
➤ Aim for win-win.

Sometimes, no matter how effective the strategies are, the other person may choose not to resolve the conflict. If so, ask yourself whether the conflict is serious enough to end the relationship? Can you live with this constant conflict? What about when it is your supervisor, colleague, superior?

If someone leaves the room angrily
➤ Do a self-analysis of the consultation: is there anything you could have done differently?
➤ Act quickly to get back in control.
➤ Be positive.
➤ Retrieve them yourself.
➤ Invite him to sit down – it is harder to be angry if you are both sitting.
➤ Think carefully.
➤ Be careful with your language: 'It would help me make a plan if knew what was on your mind' is better than 'What am I supposed to do about it?'!
➤ Indicate you are sorry for his response, that you are happy to try to find out what has happened and try to help.
➤ Try to elicit any feelings underlying the anger, for example, hopelessness, despair, chronic pain.
➤ Make good eye contact, look away briefly before replying to show you are considering your response, then glance down to allow space for his reply.
➤ Attend: lean forward, unfold your arms.
➤ Do not interrupt: let him tell the story as it helps to diffuse the anger.
➤ Actively listen and check understanding.
➤ Ask what his preferred outcome would be.
➤ Offer an expression of regret.
➤ Say what you are going to do, then do it.

Your own employers will have a policy on this, but if the angry client is on the phone, try asking them to slow down so you can write down what they are saying – thus bringing them back into a more reasonable space. If necessary, remain silent: avoid giving feedback until the anger is vented. If you can, take control back – reflect back what they are saying, and summarise your response. If none of this works, tell them you are not going to continue the conversation and then withdraw – hang up.

Strategies to reduce aggression in waiting and reception areas

Waiting is difficult. We are all busy people and would no doubt prefer to be somewhere else. It is even more difficult when waiting for important test results, if in pain, or if responsible for noisy or disruptive children. It is important for staff to identify, understand and allow for the stresses that arise while waiting to see a doctor or nurse.

Crawford, a psychotherapist at the Tavistock Clinic, London, has noted the importance too of looking at any problems in the waiting area as a symptom of wider conflicts in our organisation.[12] There are loyalties, favourites, alliances and allegiances in the relationships within all organisations and teams and the patients to consider. Because of this, it is important for provision to be made for all staff to look at the feelings stirred in them by their contact with people. Each organisation will have its own risk management procedures, which may include physical and environmental constraints, and discreet protection measures for staff. Front-line staff will be trained in assertiveness, including customer care, risk assessment and breakaway techniques such as de-escalation skills. There will be systems for lone workers, communicating who is in and out of the building, managing high-risk situations.

Within this, your environment should be one that respects and soothes the people waiting, allowing as much informal personal contact as possible. The more obvious the barriers and protective systems that are in place, the more likely the organisation is to inflame and irritate. For example, reception barriers should be low and accessible, without screens, and seating arrangements should be informal, not rigid lines.

Managing your own anger at work

If you find yourself being overly aggressive, irritable and angry with people, you are obviously stressed, and clearly not coping. We have seen that, for a variety of reasons, anger can be the most seductive of human emotions – a self-righteous monologue propels it along. In a work environment it has to be controlled, for the sake of your own professionalism and sanity and out of respect for others' feelings. The following points will help you manage it.

---

12 Crawford N. *The Psychology of Waiting and Reception in the Surgery.* Management in Medicine Conference; 1985.

Achieve control

➤ Know the warning signs: heat, wanting to shout, tears, tight chest.

➤ Count to 10.

➤ Do not vent but employ quick relaxation techniques to relieve the tension and anxiety: inhale deeply, do some isometric exercises.

➤ Decrease your volume.

➤ Monitor your thoughts and words.

➤ Focus on the facts.

➤ Remark about the situation not the person.

What you want is to change your habitual behaviour pattern and reframe your attitude. Does how you are behaving match how you want to be seen? Look at the reality. Channel the energy constructively: find your passion against injustice, for example, and work with this. Practice positive self-talk and think of new constructive responses.

In a series of studies, Gottman has documented the value of a slow start up when discussing potentially upsetting matters with another person.[13] Rapid, abrupt actions trigger alarms in the other person's sympathetic nervous system, which shake a relationship up alarmingly. If conflict is anticipated, prepare yourself, and pre-warn your partner – check it is a good time to talk, highlighting the topic, beforehand. Or try Rosenburg's[14] recommendations for non-violent communication: 'When X happens ... I feel Y ... So I need Z.' Hanson, and Mendius[15] recommend that we stay principled: doing the 'right' thing draws on both your head and your heart. Your pre-frontal cortex forms values, makes plans and instructs the rest of the brain. Your limbic system (heart) fuels the inner strength you need to pair the logical side with heart-centred and ethical virtues such as courage, generosity and forgiveness. Then you are ready to speak your truth with good intention, in a way that is beneficial, timely and expressed without harshness or malice. Afterwards, you feel good about yourself as you have acted in a way that did not add reactivity to a tense situation.

Being assertive does not always work: it does not mean that you will always get what you want. Some people might meet your assertion with aggression. Before you respond, you may decide the situation is not worth your time and energy. Decide whether you need to let things go, as you may be wiser simply to not respond. Remember, others have the right to behave badly, and you have the right to remove yourself from them rather than responding in kind.

---

13 Gottman J. *Why Marriages Succeed or Fail: and how you can make yours last*. Simon and Schuster; 1995.

14 Rosenburg M. *Nonviolent Communication: a language of life*. 2nd ed. Puddledancer Press; 2008.

15 Hanson R, Mendius R. *Buddha's Brain: the practical neuroscience of happiness, love and wisdom*. New Harbinger Publications; 2009. pp. 145–9.

KEY POINTS

➤ Conflict resolution is not about breakaway techniques, but about models of communication and how to de-escalate, diffuse or resolve conflict.

➤ It is harder to feel conflicted when we understand ourselves fully, are open and honest with ourselves and others, and recognise and accept differences between individuals and groups, in terms of values, perceptions, expectations and needs.

➤ If we provide suitable ways in which people can express their feelings about things, and ensure that we learn from previous conflicts that have been resolved, we will go a long way to living harmoniously.

➤ Conflict occurs where there are opposed principles, incompatibility: when we do not share the same values. Anger is engendered by our expectation of unacceptable behaviour on the part of others.

➤ Our attitudes and behaviour are shaped by our experiences, beliefs, our own needs and values, socio-economic variances, and the attitudes of others towards us. Thus, there will always be a mismatch between what each of us considers acceptable behaviour. The aim is to try to understand each other's world and find common ground.

➤ If we are frightened of anger, we may react in defensive ways: we ignore, placate or comply, we become over-knowledgeable and over-control through comment or behaviour.

➤ To help you understand your own responses a little more, look for recurring patterns in your life.

➤ Help to avoid anger by adopting a more relaxed and positive approach to people, being more appreciative and positive in your relationships. Build understanding and respect into your relationships. Stop blaming others for failing to meet your own ideals. Avoid negativity. Be proactive not reactive, and describe instead of interpreting. A respect for life, people and other approaches goes a long way.

➤ The most common complaints needing resolution are with poor communication; inappropriate or ineffective care management; or the complainer having some association with grief, or delayed or failed diagnosis. When this happens, the role of the manager is not to ignore, but to pull together the evidence and present it back to his or her team so that it can inform future, better practice.

➤ It is crucial to acknowledge, explain and apologise immediately if you are in the wrong. If your client is frightened or not fully competent, they need you to take charge. If they are deeply distressed, be clear, direct and honest, and keep checking that you have been understood. If they are defensive, avoid control, blame, judgement, indifference and misinformation. If the client is a chronic complainer, ask for co-operation, use positive language and take control.

➤ People who behave reactively are out of control – they are responding to external influences. These reactive responses are related to insecurity, unmet needs and fear, so these feelings can be negated by asking 'How secure do you feel here?', 'Are you getting what you need from us?', or 'What are you scared of?'.

➤ If we have a good self-image, and self-esteem, we are able to think kindly of ourselves: 'I am someone who is thoughtful, caring, who has integrity.' Not everyone is able to do this. If focussed on ego, we behave arrogantly, greedily, competitively and in a self-focussed way.

➤ Stay principled: doing the 'right' thing draws on both your head and your heart. Then you are ready to speak your truth with good intention, in a way that is beneficial, timely, and expressed without harshness or malice.

FURTHER READING

Benjamin S. *Perfect Phrases for Dealing with Difficult People: hundreds of ready-to-use phrases for handling conflict, confrontations and challenging personalities*. McGraw-Hill Professional; 2007.

Kirschner R. *Dealing with Difficult People UK Edition: 24 lessons for bringing out the best in everyone*. US Adaptations; 2007.

Lavelle J. *Water Off a Duck's Back: how to deal with frustrating situations, awkward, exasperating and manipulative people and … keep smiling!*. Blue Ice Publishing; 2010.

Lilley R. *Dealing with Difficult People (creating success)*. Kogan Page; 2010.

Lindenfield G. *Managing Anger: simple steps to dealing with frustration and threat*. Thorsons; 2000.

Section 3

Clinical challenges

CHAPTER 10

Setting the boundaries

What is more important to you as a practitioner: that your own patient/client gets his or her course of treatment; or that all those waiting get seen? Is it more important to you to feel liked, or do you find it easy to be assertive and hold a boundary? Do you consider it is better for you to remain available to the patient in case they need your help, or are you most likely to feel satisfied when they are up and running and you can withdraw your care? Do you like to feel needed? Have you fully considered the client's needs (not yours!) and considered whether you are the right person to meet those needs? Whose agenda are we meeting when we take on a new patient, a new duty of care?

This section begins to explore the management of tensions. They present as something we have to balance daily in all our services, as we are employed to work within a system where budget cuts bite and new ways of working more efficiently and effectively are developed. Part of our clinical development is to learn to manage these tensions, so that we feel comfortable that the service we deliver is the best it can possibly be for the greatest number of people. As public services, we have a fundamental duty to do the most good and the least harm for the most number of people within the resources available. Frameworks such as Malcomess's Care Aims,[1] and the diligent use of goal setting[2] have provided tools to measure the input required more fairly to reduce the impact of pathology within the general population. The only equitable way of doing this is by working out who is most at risk in the population we serve and which of those people we can help the most. How can this be achieved? How can we feel comfortable with discharging people back into the care of others, with whom we may share professional rivalries? How do we know our decision making is perfect? Do we feel comfortable managing the risk?

I would argue that clinically, morally and professionally, we have a commitment to the NHS to deliver the care that is required to the very best standard, and to ensure that care is delivered efficiently, effectively and at the best price. In the following chapters, we explore these values and examine the ways by which we as clinicians can contribute to the clinical effectiveness

1 www.careaims.com (accessed April 2013).
2 Simpson S, Sparkes C. Goal negotiation (3). *Speech and Language Therapy in Practice*. 2001. Available at: www.intandem.co.uk (accessed April 2013).

agenda. We are required to do so morally, by our employers, and by our professional bodies.[3] Managers in the NHS manage the demand by managing the referral boundary, ensuring capacity while remaining faithful to the core principles of equity and fairness. They also collect and produce data that supports the evidence for working in particular ways, and ensure that outcome and throughput remain balanced. For us clinicians to work effectively, we need to support management in creating clear boundaries: for our public, ourselves, our profession, the NHS. We need to communicate these boundaries clearly, confidently and respectfully. We need to discuss expectations with those we work with, so that they are prepared – forewarned – about the limits of any treatment so that expectations are not raised unnecessarily. People need clear, unbiased information about the clinical role and the treatment trajectory, and the clinician's specific role in this. For this, we need to be assertive.

Users of our services will have different expectations of services offered, which are influenced by factors such as their own cultural and family models of healthcare and ways of managing their own health, previous use of services, and perceptions of illness severity. There will be differing levels of expectation around what is fair and realistic, and this needs to be managed carefully.

We know our services cannot be all things to all people. They are funded entirely out of the public purse, and so all of us working within it are accountable for the taxpayer's money, to ensure that it is well spent. Successive governments have brought in various measures to ensure that this money can be accounted for, and that the spend is seen to be prudent and fair. This is against the backdrop of public expectation that health and social care will give whatever care is needed for as long as is needed, so once clinicians start discussing the fact no more help is forthcoming (or needed), they are often disbelieved. There is also a healthy debate emerging among doctors which highlights growing evidence that modern medicine is causing harm through ever earlier detection and 'even wider definition' of disease,[4] resulting in even more (perhaps unnecessary) treatment and a certain increase in worry among those found to have some early or mild evidence of disease, and some over-diagnosis of pathology, all generating a rise in public expectation.

Clinicians need to have much more intelligent, thought-provoking discussions with their public and set clear boundaries about what is on offer from the very beginning. Clinicians, not just managers, need to take

---

3 Health Professions Council. *Standards of Proficiency*. Health Professions Council; 2007. Health Professions Council. *Standards of Conduct, Performance and Ethics*. Health Professions Council; 2008. Available at: www.hpc-uk.org/assets/documents (accessed April 2013). Body R, McAllister L. *Ethics in Speech and Language Therapy*. Wiley-Blackwell; 2009.

4 Preventing overdiagnosis: how to stop harming the healthy. *BMJ*. 2012 May 30. Cited in: Porter M. Body and soulhealth. *The Times*. 2012 Jun 5. Spence D. The advance of modern psychiatry. *BMJ*. 2012 May 12.

responsibility for considering the funding realities: how can we best meet the needs of our patients and clients? We need to be seen to be working in an effective, evidence-based way, and we need to develop the kind of advanced reflective, clinical thinking in order to be taken seriously as clinicians, and to help us in our difficult discussions, especially if people are demanding a level of care that is not outcome based. A lack of resources is not an adequate reason for not taking on a patient or client, but equal access does not mean equal input.[5] In other words, we have to be able to justify our clinical decision making at all times, and we as clinicians have to take responsibility for making *all* our decisions evidenced based, and saying 'no' when we cannot help. In order to discharge this duty effectively, we need to be assertive with our management team to ensure that we obtain the necessary professional and clinical support structures, and to ensure good access to training, clinical supervision, peer review and case discussion.

Of course, there is a common and uncomfortable understanding that there has been a massive political shift in recent years away from welfare focussed and 'quality of life' healthcare delivery; from a well-being model towards a business model (which we will explore here), which many feel focuses too much on efficiencies, often at the expense of quality of care and concern with human welfare. However, we do need to run the NHS especially as a business, as the shift in demography, expense of new pharmacology and treatments necessitates, but any shift towards efficiency does not need to mean that we lose the ability to connect with one another or to value things that nourish, support and nurture all of us through life.

Our NHS values spell out our need to treat people with respect and dignity, to commit to quality of care, to improve lives with compassion, and to work inclusively, without excluding anyone or any group. But the NHS has to be more than caring. It has to be seen to meet a whole raft of national, political and social expectations. It is an expensive machine to run, and has to provide value for money, increase patient choice, improve the patient experience, reduce inequalities, work within budget, improve performance year on year and provide a platform to support public health. Healthcare organisations are expected to:

➤ apply the principles of sound clinical and corporate governance
➤ actively support all employees to promote openness, honesty, probity, accountability, and the economic, efficient and effective use of resources
➤ undertake systematic risk assessment and risk management

---

5 Malcomess K. The Care Aims model in speech and language therapy. In: Anderson C, van der Gaag A, editors. *Speech and Language Therapy: issues in professional practice*. Whurr Publishers Ltd; 2005. Ch. 4, pp. 43–71.

➤ ensure financial management achieves economy, effectiveness, efficiency, probity and accountability in the use of resources
➤ challenge discrimination, promote equality and respect human rights,[6]

in addition to providing safe, effective and innovative care.[7]

In this section we investigate the different ways in which the applications of boundaries impact on our work: how national and professional clinical standards necessarily constrain what we do and how we do it, and how, if at all, they limit what we can and cannot deliver. The second consideration is more personal – as NHS workers, we sign up to upholding the values of the organisation we represent, and all too often as clinicians we forget this, narrowing our beam of focus onto patient care only. Of course, this focus is crucial, but it need not be absolute, and good clinicians can work within a strategic framework too. In terms of assertiveness, it is important that we understand and absorb some of these wider NHS values and develop an ease in communicating some of them to our patients, who may need gently to be brought into a different way of looking at their NHS, and the need for them to incorporate some level of responsibility to contribute to their own healthcare rather than simply be a passive, dependent recipient of that care.

SOME PRINCIPLES

This rapid pace of change can itself be placed within the broader context of the public management restructuring of health, education and social services that has been taking place in the UK since the 1980s. This restructuring has been introduced and maintained by successive governments with a view to making public services more efficient, accountable and responsive to 'customer' need.[8] Many have argued that this restructuring has also aimed to make professional practice more transparent and controllable. Others[9] argue that private sector notions of market forces, assessment and management have underpinned the rise of 'managerialism', audit culture and 'neo-bureaucracy' in public sector services, where economic rationalism and technicism, efficiency, accountability

6 Department of Health. *Standards for Better Health*. Department of Health; 2006. Available at: www.dh.gov.uk (accessed April 2013).
7 Kennedy I. *State of Healthcare 2008*. Healthcare Commission; 2008.
8 Rizq R. Public sector practice: IAPT, anxiety and envy: a psychoanalytic view of NHS primary care mental health services today. *British Journal of Psychotherapy*. 2011; **27**(1): 37–55.
9 Loewenthal D. The nature of psychotherapeutic knowledge: psychotherapy and counselling in universities [editorial]. *European Journal of Psychotherapy, Counselling and Health*. 2002; **5**(4): 331–46. Harrison S, Smith C. Neo-bureaucracy and public management: The case of medicine in the National Health Service. *Competition and Change*. 2003; **7**(4): 243–54.

and performativity are privileged over basic trust in public sector professionals.[10] These political tensions are explicit, and demonstrable in and among both NHS workers and external stakeholders.

Meeting clinical standards

There are various drivers set as quality standards by the government and, although constantly changing, current standards have their roots in some concepts set earlier in the NHS history. The idea of clinical governance, for example, was introduced within the NHS in the early 1980s, with an aim to bring together all of the components of good clinical practice and quality and to arrange to measure and monitor them. It aimed to improve patient care through achieving high standards, reflective practice and risk management, as well as personal and professional development. The concept has grown and is now embedded in NHS thinking.

Maxwell applied the ideas of *total quality management* (TQM) to the NHS in 1984.[11] TQM is an integrative philosophy of management for continuously improving the quality of products and processes. It functions on the premise that the quality of products and processes is the responsibility of everyone who is involved with the creation or consumption of the products or services offered by an organisation. As a management tool in healthcare, TQM aims to capitalise on the involvement of management, workforce, suppliers and clients/ patients, in order to meet or exceed 'customer' expectations, by incorporating cross-functional product design, efficient process management, supplier quality management, patient involvement, information and feedback, committed leadership, strategic planning, cross-functional training, and employee involvement.[12] The concept is about reducing risk by constantly improving the product you are offering in relation to the customer's needs.

The NHS is a not for profit organisation, so we need to revisit what quality means in that context. It may be fair to say that quality in healthcare has to provide:

➤ value for money
➤ fitness for purpose
➤ customer satisfaction.

---

10 O'Neill O. *A Question of Trust*. Cambridge University Press; 2002. Orbach S. Democratizing psychoanalysis. *European Journal of Psychotherapy and Counselling*. 2007; 9(1): 7–21. Phillips A. *Equals*. Fontana; 2002. Power M. *The Audit Society: rituals of verification*. Oxford University Press; 1997.
11 Maxwell RJ. Perspectives in NHS management: quality assessment in health. *BMJ*. 1984; **288**: 1470–2.
12 Brooks T. Total quality management in the NHS. *Health Service Management*. 1992; **88**(2): 17–19. Source: King's Fund Centre.

We need be acknowledge that we an part of an organisation in pursuit of continuous improvement, an approach which focuses on the patient, and to understand that the organisation exists to meet the needs of the patient, not itself.

When commissioning services, the NHS today ensures it meets certain standards, set down and enforced through audit by the *Care Quality Commission*. In the 1990s, a 'Gold Standard' service had to meet performance assessment framework markers, all of which would still apply today in the new GP commissioning world.

➤ **Accessible:** no physical, cultural or linguistic barriers, timely.
➤ **Appropriate:** conforms to legislation, researched based, meets needs of the population.
➤ **Effective:** promotes health and recovery, research based, national service frameworks guidelines followed.
➤ **Efficient:** best use resources, skills, money, people, buildings, equipment.
➤ **Equitable:** respectful to all, service provided on basis of need not personal characteristics.
➤ **Relevant:** responsive to the population served; sufficient, balanced, gaps.
➤ **Acceptable:** does it meet the cultural and religious expectations of the users?
➤ **Knowledge based:** does sound and accurate information support decision making?
➤ **Accountable:** principally and financially, is the care outcome based?
➤ **Integrative:** involves other agencies.

TQM does not supplant traditional approaches; it simply provides the tools with which traditional medical knowledge can be made to work better.

➤ It is concerned with achieving value for money and using resources effectively.
➤ It gives workers more opportunity to contribute to the development of services.
➤ It changes the culture of an organisation to achieve tangible benefits for everyone.
➤ It fails when the leaders are uncommitted or suppress desires for improvement.
➤ It aims not just to satisfy the needs of the patient, but to delight them.
➤ It aims for continuous improvement, not just front of house.
➤ It harnesses conflict and focuses on improving processes.
➤ It seeks to reduce inter-professional wrangling.
➤ It does not just improve numbers, but also improves services.

➤ It is involved with improvement not punishment – if your patients require more expensive care because they are older and more fragile, this a is fine and defensible position.[13]

These concepts have continually evolved, and the *Common Assessment Framework* (CAF) is now the current common European quality management instrument for the public sector. It is a free tool to assist public sector organisations in improving their performance. The CAF helps the organisations to perform a self-assessment with the involvement of all staff, to develop an improvement plan based on the results of the self-assessment and to implement the improvement actions. The model is based on the premise that excellent results in organisational performance, citizens/customers, people and society are achieved through leadership driving strategy and planning, people, partnerships and resources, and processes. It looks at the organisation from different angles at the same time – the holistic approach of organisation performance analysis. It looks very familiar. The CAF principles of excellence are:

➤ results orientation
➤ citizen/customer focus
➤ leadership and constancy of purpose
➤ management of processes and facts
➤ involvement of people
➤ continuous improvement and innovation
➤ mutually beneficial partnerships
➤ corporate social responsibility.[14]

Every time we devise a new clinical pathway or research a new clinical tool, we need to bring awareness of these standards into our work. The standards incorporate the clinical governance standards discussed earlier: development of any activities that improve service quality, continuous identification and management of risk, and continuing professional development of staff.

The principles of clinical governance help us to ensure good practice within the NHS:

➤ co-operating and working with others
➤ applying the principles locally, to your practice
➤ focussing on improving and maintaining high standards of care
➤ setting clear service standards

---

13 Cua KO, McKone KE, Schroeder RG. Relationships between implementation of TQM, JIT, and TPM and manufacturing performance. *Journal of Operations Management.* 2001; **19**(6): 675–94.
14 CAF Resource Centre. *CAF External Feedback.* European Institute of Public Administration; 2010. p. 64. McCormick JS. Effectiveness and efficiency. *JRCGP.* 1981; **31**: 299–302.

➤ performing clinical audit
➤ ensuring evidence-based practices are carried out
➤ collecting records to help review performance and monitor patient care
➤ implementing risk management plans
➤ reporting adverse healthcare incidents
➤ setting clear performance standards for all staff
➤ promoting a learning environment
➤ valuing openness
➤ involving the public.

To ensure that we all work to develop clinical standards, the systems embraced by clinical governance include clinical audit, risk management, revalidation, all evidence-based clinical practice (NICE, national/regional protocols and local guidance), audit of consumer feedback and accreditation.

GPs, running as small businesses, foundation trusts and all provider services are crucially aware of the emerging tensions between equality/choice, demand/ resources and efficiency/quality, and managing these tensions is crucial. There will always be a major tension between providing the very best clinical care and the cost of that care. And practising the very best medicine at all times is impossible – the aim must always be to minimise the risk of harm. Various clinical tools have been developed to help us do so: one is for us to ensure our practice is evidence based.

Evidence-based practice (EBP)

EBP is changing the way we all practise. In the current environment, it is not sufficient to rely solely on what we learnt at university and have picked up along the way since then – although there is an obvious requirement to demonstrate continual learning and development. The stakeholders we now report to ask us to justify how we provide treatment to our patients, and using EBP provides us with real and solid reasons for providing the services we select.

Using EBP means giving the best possible care to our clients and letting go of old or ineffective practices when a different way is possible and effective. It means choosing client-focussed service delivery and being able to explain why we work in this way rather than being compelled to use budget-conscious service delivery because we cannot prove our treatments are effective.[15] There are many professionals –specific sites, as above – which assist us in our quest for EBD. Some are included in the Further reading section at the end of the chapter.

---

15 BITE. Speech. Available at: www.speechbite.com.au/ebp.php (accessed April 2013).

In the mid-1990s, the Department of Health[16] adapted Roth and Fonagy's principles,[17] originally applied to psychotherapy research, and produced a four-step model for improved patient care. This model can be used reliably for any service provision:

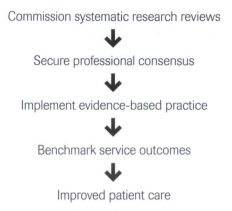

Commission systematic research reviews

⬇

Secure professional consensus

⬇

Implement evidence-based practice

⬇

Benchmark service outcomes

⬇

Improved patient care

We have many umbrella supports for the services we deliver, and all of these are relevant for both primary (community) and tertiary (secondary) care services. I feel it is our clinical responsibility to understand how these organisations work to support our decision making, to ensure we work to the standards set and to give our public support to the principles they advocate. Too often we collude with the public and the media in their distrust of these organisations, giving the implication that we too feel there is a limitless pot of public money that should be spent entirely on the part of the service we represent! We need a more balanced, measured and strategic understanding of the tensions involved. This does not mean that we cannot fight for our corner, but that we have to be seen to understand the broader implications of what we fight for.

Here are some broad pointers to some of these organisations.

National Institute for Health and Care Excellence (NICE)

What does NICE actually do?
NICE appraises what is considered to be the best interventions and treatments and produces guidelines to ensure a faster, more uniform uptake of treatments which work best for patients.

---

16 Department of Health. *Creating a Patient-led NHS: delivering the NHS improvement plan.* Department of Health; 2005. Department of Health. *IAPT Key Performance Indicators: revised guidance.* Department of Health; 2009.
17 Roth A, Fonagy P. *What Works for Whom? A critical review of psychotherapy research.* The Guilford Press; 1996.

NICE is one strand of clinical governance. The team offers authoritative guidance on the highest standards of care. It aims to improve the nature and completeness of data held in general practice through appraising technology, developing clinical care programmes and promoting the monitoring of clinical performance through:

➤ audit
➤ referral protocols
➤ procedural manuals
➤ nursing benchmarks
➤ disease management protocols
➤ integrated care pathways,

and clinical guidelines that are multidisciplinary, formally evidenced, clinical and cost-effective and applicable to the majority. Given we are scientists working in a scientific arena, it is seems odd that many clinicians are angry with some of the NICE decisions. Again, this represents parochial, not strategic thinking. To feel comfortable with our broader responsibilities, we need to go beyond having only a limited or narrow outlook, the focus on our own service, and instead fight for the whole NHS.

National service frameworks (NSFs)[18] were policies originally set by the NHS in England in the 1990s to define standards of care for major medical issues such as cancer, coronary heart disease, mental health and diabetes. NSFs are also defined for some key patient groups, including children and older people. They set clear quality requirements for care, based on the best available evidence of what treatments and services work most effectively for patients. One of the main strengths of each strategy is that it is inclusive, having been developed in partnership with health professionals, patients, carers, health service managers, voluntary agencies and other experts. Implementation of NSF's were identified as one of the Saving Lives priorities in the National Priorities Guidance for 2000/01 to 20002/03. From that point on, all NHS bodies have been expected to work with their local communities to take the guidance forward.

The two main roles of NSFs are:

➤ to set clear quality requirements for care based on the best available evidence of what treatments and services work most effectively for patients
➤ to offer strategies and support to help organisations achieve these.

NSFs establish models of treatment and care based on evidence of best practice. They look for uniformity of treatment to a minimum standard and consistency across major care areas. They provide a treatment framework for a particular disorder or group of diseases. Broadly, they aim to address:

---

18 www.nhs.uk/NHSEngland/NSF (accessed April 2013).

➤ healthcare improvements
➤ inequalities of access
➤ differences of outlook
➤ differences of outcome
➤ differences in quality of care
➤ post code rationing.

Specifically, NSFs set standards/benchmarks for best care. They are set up in collaboration with relevant professional bodies and link with NHS research and development centres. They address Care Pathways – the programme of care from primary through to tertiary and secondary care. They include primary/secondary care prevention and rehabilitation strands. Within this, they look at managerial, clinical and technical/technical change, for example, referral advice, triage, direct booking systems – anything that results in fewer patients being seen with faster, more convenient access.

An example of an early coronary heart disease NSF

The coronary heart disease NSF[19] was the first framework to be introduced into general practice universally in the early 2000s.

The following data is collected from patients on a GP list:

➤ diagnosis of coronary heart disease
➤ diagnosis of transient ischaemic attack/ischaemic stroke
➤ diagnosis of peripheral vascular disease
➤ blood pressure recording
➤ blood pressure control
➤ lipid levels
➤ diabetes
➤ smoking status
➤ relevant lifestyle factors
➤ number prescribed nitrates, beta-blockers, ACE inhibitors or aspirin.

This information is collected, sorted and managed, which demonstrates why managers need clinical support within their team for the process. It is fashionable to dismiss public sector managers as representing the non-caring side of clinical practice, focussed solely on resource management. Managers are often criticised for restricting clinical decision making, preventing innovation and curtailing clinical freedom. However, demonstrably, managers have a crucial role to play in ensuring service equity, patient access and healthcare improvements. Managers

---

19 Department of Health. *National Service Framework for Coronary Heart Disease*. HSC 2000/012. Department of Health; 2000.

have an unenviable task managing these tensions and keeping the public, the government and the clinicians happy. In our NSF example, it is the managers who ensure that the practice team not only sees patients face to face (which is what the face of the NHS provides) but also ensures that the team:

➤ meets as a clinical team every quarter
➤ has an agreed protocol for the assessment, treatment and follow-up of patients with cardiovascular disease
➤ arranges to see patients in an appointment that gives time to cover the areas required by the NSF
➤ knows the number and proportion of patients with a diagnosis of heart failure
➤ keeps the medical records in date order
➤ has drug information readily discernible on its medical records.

Who within the organisation is going to manage this process? The managers. The clinicians will assess, give advice and prescribe, but it is the managers who set up and manage the recall process, who manage the audit process, who are responsible for controls assurance, who check there is a procedure in place to identify and manage clinical risk, and who ensure there is a method of reporting adverse healthcare event. Healthcare managers are there to assist and encourage the development of leadership skills and knowledge among clinicians. It is part of their job to:

➤ develop the appropriate accountability structures
➤ integrate continuing professional development into quality improvement programmes
➤ encourage and develop more formal links between primary and secondary care
➤ implement evidence-based practice
➤ support and develop the clinical information infrastructure
➤ ensure that changing practice occurs in the light of audit, research, complaints and risk management
➤ develop the mechanisms to ensure that clinical audit is integrated into the organisation to assist and support the development of multidisciplinary and interagency working.

User involvement

User involvement is a major area of significant change, and one that we will address again in this section. We have seen that since in early 1990s, service users have been reconfigured as consumers, and as such have of necessity, and rightly, been encouraged to be more involved with service configuration. There has been a range of government policies to support this principle,[20] which has led to the various models previously discussed, including client-centred care, public/patient partnerships, shared decision making. This paradigm cultural shift has required time, commitment, courage and reflection. Both users and clinicians require 'confidence, competence, time, resources and [the] appropriate tools to engage in meaningful dialogue about working partnerships'.[21]

There is no doubt that the clinical governance agenda and, in particular, user involvement does support a broader, positive and more inclusive approach to healthcare provision. Perhaps we too need some public recognition for the management teams working behind the scenes to ensure these clinical governance challenges are met. Clinicians are challenged by the extra work involved in setting up and maintaining the systems required and supporting the clinical standards set, but we all have a role in encouraging sharing of good practice, to assist others and support the principle of standards, to voice concerns when poor practice is noted, and to provide good clinical leadership so that evidence, outcome-based practices are developed and shared.

REFLECTIVE PRACTICE

In order to clarify our thinking, decision making and to strengthen our evidence-based practice – to make sure we are working to the agenda set for us – we as clinicians need to reflect constantly on our practice. Most of us, when working, actively interpret, evaluate and make conclusions based on what we have considered, based on our prior knowledge and experience: we reflect on and analyse events to give them a narrative that we feel comfortable with. If this reflection is not now part of our working lives, it does need to be. It needs to be made a 'purposeful and strategic process'[22] that underpins and drives the maintenance of our professional competence. As with the audit cycle, it demands a commitment to action following the process. Each profession carries its own demand: The Health Professionals Council Standards of Proficiency has its own:

---

20 Department of Health. *Involving Patients and the Public in Healthcare*. Department of Health; 2001. Department of Health. *The Expert Patient*. Department of Health; 2001. Department of Health. *The NHS Improvement Plan: putting people at the heart of public services*. Department of Health; 2004.

21 Swinburn K. Journeys with aphasia, personal reflection. In: Anderson C, van der Gaag A, editors. *Speech and Language Therapy: issues in professional practice*. Whurr Publishers Ltd; 2005. Ch. 7, p. 116.

22 Eyles J, Giles D, Schmiede A. Cited in: Ash SL, Clayton PH. Generating, deepening, and documenting learning: the power of critical reflection in applied learning. *Journal of Applied Learning in Higher Education*. 2009; 1(1): 25–48.

'Registrants must be able to audit, reflect on and review practice: understand the value of reflection on practice and record the outcome of such reflection.'[23]

Why we reflect can range from:
➤ meeting our professional requirements
➤ engaging critically with issues at work
➤ identifying potential areas for change within our service
➤ identifying potential areas for change within our profession or practice
➤ an (inherent) desire to develop our professional knowledge, skills and understanding.[24]

In order to develop professionally, we need actively to notice what we are doing, and to be able to articulate and explain our choices and evaluate whether our experience adds to, confirms, or challenges current practice, research and thinking. It is through the process of challenging current practice that new ideas, knowledge and theory develop; the process enables us to respond to critical challenges set by the public, management or a court of law.

It is only through reflective practice we can explore our core values and fully integrate our experiences. McGormick[25] adds that it provides a way again for us to:
➤ work out how to improve our practice
➤ bring the multiple demands and clinical complexities of our work into the open
➤ explore issues of challenge and stress, personal growth and development
➤ deal with difficult issues of handling interpersonal conflict
➤ receive affirmation and encouragement.

Reflection is a useful way of examining your own work experiences. At is simplest level, it supports you to question those experiences and through this examination gain a deeper understanding of both your role and your ability to perform effectively at work. Reflective practice aids both personal and professional development, and enables us to further our clinical thinking. The practice hopefully develops the capacity to reflect in action, to think on your feet. Reflective thinking is a type of problem solving, where our feelings about the process are central to the analysis. It is where we 're-frame' the experience as a way of resolving both the problem and the difficult feelings associated with

---

23 Health Professions Council. *Standards of Proficiency*. Health Professions Council; 2007. Health Professions Council. *Standards of Conduct, Performance and Ethics*. Health Professions Council; 2007.
24 McCormick M. Reflection, we all do it. *RCSLT Bulletin*. 2012 Jun. pp. 24–5.
25 Ibid.

it, and move on with the experience.[26] It is important to reiterate that reflection is not rumination or rehearsal of the same narrative, experience or feeling. This we all do – it is tempting and easy, but it is cyclical and does not further our thinking and allow for analysis and change to occur.

Some models of reflection

There are several recommended models of reflective practice, some simple and some more complex. Kolb has written about learning being holistic and adaptive, a continuous lifelong process.[27] These models reflect this way of thinking.

Model 1

Description: what happened?

⬇

How did you feel?

⬇

Evaluation/analysis: what was good and bad about the situation and why?

⬇

Conclusion/action: anything else you could have done? What will you do in the future?

Model 2

The Lewinian Learning cycle.

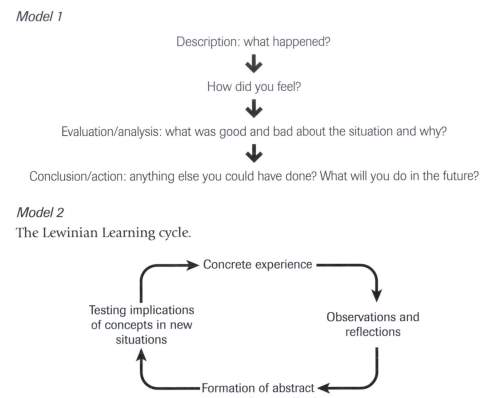

Figure 10.1   The Lewinian experimental learning model (source: Kolb DA. *Experiential Learning: experience as the source of learning and development.* Prentice Hall; 1984. p. 21)

---

26 Schon D. *The Reflective Practitioner: how professionals think in action.* Temple Smith; 1983.
27 Kolb DA. *Experiential Learning: experience as the source of learning and development.* Prentice Hall; 1984.

Model 3

This more complex model includes the use of creative and problem solving skills.

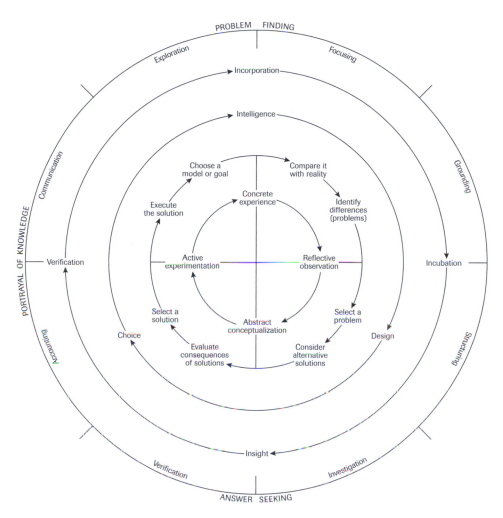

Figure 10.2 Similarities among conceptions of basic adaptive processes: inquiry/research, creativity, decision making, problem solving, learning (source: Kolb DA. *Experiential Learning: experience as the source of learning and development.* Prentice Hall; 1984. p. 33)

Even more complex models have arisen since these early works.[28] These models tend to concentrate more on the need to develop our self-awareness and

28 Atkins S, Murphy K. Reflective practice. *Nursing Standard.* 1994; **8**(39): 49–56. Johns C, Graham J. Using a reflective model of nursing and guided reflection. *Nursing Standard.* 1996; **11**(2): 34–8.

support our journey towards advanced clinical thinking. Here, the reflection is orientated towards the development of a kind of practical wisdom. It is through our awareness of uncomfortable thoughts and feelings – a creative tension – that we develop a need to unpick the dilemmas. It is through the consideration of the perspective of different people within the experience that the learning occurs. We learn to work out whether our feelings are prompted by personal, professional or organisational interests. We learn to gain perspective, and analyse and challenge the experience from above: were there any key or recurring features? Are there any assumptions to challenge? Are there any alternative actions to consider? We learn to evaluate the relevance of our knowledge and understand if it helps to explain or solve the problem. It is through this process that learning occurs and new, and different, actions arise. It is not simply a cognitive process – emotions are central to all learning. The practice is forcing us to question what it is that we know and how we come to know it.

Some of the core attributes needed to develop advanced communication skills and developed clinical thinking are the development of practical wisdom; reflexivity (the reviewing of our self-development over time); mindfulness (seeking congruence between our logical, emotional and practical sides); a commitment to learning (curiosity, openness, non-defensiveness); understanding of self and others; empathy; and the empowerment needed to take action based on the insights gained.

Nurses have been using models of reflective practice since the early 1990s.[29] Here is one model, useful to all professions.

Description
Describe the situation and the key issues.

Reflection
➤ How was I feeling? What made me feel like that? Was a button pressed? Which one?
➤ What was I trying to achieve? Consider the purpose and meaning of your actions.
➤ Did I respond effectively? This cue penetrates and brings to light any contradiction between our actions and values.
➤ Were there consequences of my actions on myself and others, and what were they?
➤ How were the others feeling and why?

---

29 Johns, Graham, note 28 above.

Influencing factors

Internal and external factors.

➤ What factors influences the way I was thinking, feeling, responding? Expectations from self or others? Values? Theory? Emotional entanglement? Limited skills? Passive/stressed/time? Misplaced concern or loyalty? Fears of sanction?

➤ What knowledge did or might have helped inform me? If an organisational response is required, use knowledge of any protocols, etc.

➤ Did I act in tune with my values, the ethical basis of my practice?

Alternative strategies

Any other choices and their consequences.

Learning

➤ Could I have dealt better with the situation?

➤ How has this experience changed my way of knowing in practice?

➤ What am I doing as a result of this experience.

ADVANCED REFLECTIVE THINKING

The application of reflective practice is apparent when we plan care for our patients and clients at a macro (strategic) and micro (local) level, in both the overall delivery of care and the care planning process applied to individual patients and clients. This is best illustrated by looking at one process, Care Aims. Care Aims is a philosophy of care that is taught by Kate Malcomess,[30] which can be applied across all professional groups in health and social care. One of the most important principles from Care Aims teaching is the support and development of advanced reflective clinical thinking. The model does represent a challenge, a fundamental shift in traditional clinical thinking, and because of this Malcomess quite rightly recommends her full training[31] so that the concepts are completely understood, to avoid struggle with the core principles of the model. Again, this level of thinking challenges us personally and professionally, and its application requires a high level of thinking, planning, reflection and assertiveness skills.

As we saw at the beginning of this chapter, one of our aims in working with people to clarify who is most at risk in our population and who we can help the most. Each NHS trust has safeguarding policies that reinforce the concept. It is also about making sure we only hold a solid duty of care for those whom we can help the most. Malcomess reinforces the concept of 'levels' of care, set by the Department of Health. The education sector, too, is now working using

---

30 Malcomess, note 5 above.
31 www.careaims.com (accessed April 2013).

terminology that discusses particular levels, or 'waves' of care: terms that are used interchangeably. Here we look at how the terms work in the provision of clinical services within the NHS. At the first level there is self, or public help – where no intervention is required from statutory services. Then various levels of support are prescribed.

Wave 1: Universal services.
Wave 2: Targeted services.
Wave 3: Specialist services.
Wave 4: Regional services.

At the level of wave 1 and 2 we are concerned in the NHS with general health promotion, prevention, identification and signposting. By offering services at waves 1 and 2 we are encouraging the public and the referrers to take responsibility whenever possible, to reduce the risk in the population. It is recommended we do this through a variety of means: telephone advice lines (NHS Direct or those run by specialist services), expert patient programmes, targeted patient group work, teaching to other health professionals, teachers and carers, etc. Our aim here is to support the tenet that prevention is better than a cure, with outcomes being better with early intervention, intervening before the condition becomes a problem.

This in turn helps to identify the people who need actual, specialist, clinical intervention at wave 3.

Autonomous clinicians responsible for assessment (and diagnosis/ treatment), nurses, doctors, therapists etc., have a duty to universal services and a statutory duty to assess. That assessment may be at triage where we determine from the information given we are given if the person's needs fit the criteria for wave 3 intervention or if they can be addressed at a more general wave 1 or 2. As the safeguarding literature notes, we do not have a statutory or legal duty to treat: the Education Act, Children's Act, Disability Discrimination Act and Mental Capacity Act do not include a duty to treat. However, if we as clinicians do decide to accept a duty of care, it must be provided. If it cannot be provided, the patient and referrers must be told why. Lack of resources is not a reason for negligence here, so once we decide and accept someone onto our caseload we are obligated to see them; we begin to hold a legal duty of care. No one else, including our managers, can make that decision for us. Because we are autonomous, we cannot plead 'higher order': autonomy is covered by common law. This means that the care we provide is of the same level as a reasonable person, at the same professional standing, would give.

It can be equally difficult to know when the duty of care stops. Once we have assessed and determined that there is a need that can be worked with. Smart working would require that we as clinicians think about what we are doing with, and to, that patient at every stage of their treatment. Who we are seeing, why we are seeing them, what are we doing, when we want to do it etc.[32]

Malcomess helps us to define more clearly the treatment plan, and encourages us to ensure that the 'episode' of care is an episode, not an ongoing, ill-considered and unplanned treatment. At the end of that episode, you reassess to see whether the goals have been achieved. Have those needs been met? Are there any other needs? Is there any indication for another episode of care?

If there is still a foreseeable risk, for example, a condition that can fluctuate without any reason, such as cystic fibrosis, stammering, arthritis, and that deems ongoing clinical intervention, that may be provided. If so, the patient can be asked to contact the service when and if a new problem occurs, instead of the service automatically setting a review. If not, the patient must be discharged. It is important to remember that when we discharge we no longer hold a duty of care. However, this means we may need to ensure that those who hold a permanent duty of care are made aware of the discharge, i.e. GP/health visitor/ consultant.

This decision-making process can only happen through constant and ongoing, circular reflection. We assess the patient/client and situation, we hypothesis about what we think the need is, we predict what we may need to change the need, we set goals and care plans, we put this intervention in place, and then we reflect again.

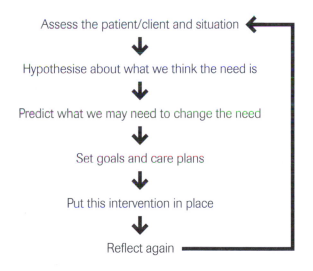

Here the reflection itself requires some advanced clinical thinking. To further this, and to consider our care to be truly patient-centred, we need to

32 Beirne P. Implementation of the Care Aims model: challenges and opportunities. In: Anderson C, van der Gaag A, editors. *Speech and Language Therapy: issues in professional practice.* Whurr Publishers Ltd; 2005. Ch. 5, pp. 72–85.

remember that the only impact we have concerns about is the impact of our intervention(s) on the patient (and their family, indirectly). Not the impact on our diary, or any other involved party – a concerned teacher, a nurse, a parent – but the impact on the needs of that patient. We may have to acknowledge there is going to be no useful impact, which is difficult when we can see there is still a problem. Professionally, clinicians have traditionally been taught that where there is a problem they have to solve it, they have to intervene, to try: the system is diagnostically driven. As Beirne describes in her critique of the Care Aims model, we can describe *what* we are doing in minute detail, but rarely ask ourselves why we are doing it.[33]

In the NHS, many services have been set up to review patients automatically, not to give the patients the power and authority to make that decision themselves.

Because of this – paternalistic – decision-making process, culturally it is hard for a parent or other interested party to give up the control and allow a consenting child or adult to take charge of their own destiny. There is no denying it is challenging to watch your child refuse to talk to their friend using their communication aid, but it is their life, not yours. It is difficult to watch someone choking because they have chosen oral nutrition not PEG feeding, fully understanding the consequences of this. Or to see an adult with COPD struggle to breathe because they have chosen to refuse further treatment. But we do need to allow consenting patients to make their own decisions, and if this is tough on us, these are concerns we need to take to our supervisors, not share with patients or their carers.

It is worth here reflecting on issues of consent. Various statutes (the Mental Capacity Act 2005, the Mental Health Acts, the Safeguarding Vulnerable Groups Act 2006, among others) caution us around the principles of consent. They clarify, reform and update legal uncertainties around decision making on behalf of others. Basically, people must be supported as much as possible to make a decision before anyone concludes that they cannot make their own decision. Any decisions made do not have to be 'rational'. People can make unwise or eccentric decisions, which may not appear to be rational to another person. Thus a decision not to have treatment, made by a consenting adult, has to be accepted by us as clinicians, even though we may not agree with the decision.

Although Care Aims may on the surface appear to be resource based, our clinical aim is not about how many people can be discharged, but an ongoing reflection about the patient's need, and whether there is an ongoing role for us. The reflection is about asking the right questions: for each episode of care, what evidence is there that I am discharging my duty of care? Discharging a duty is

---

33 Beirne, note 32 above, pp. 5, 73.

different from discharging the patient or client. It is about making sure you are doing your job, assessing if your time is being spent well and remembering that we are trying to do the most good, and least harm, to most people. Have my goals been achieved? If not, was it unrealistic or was the advice not carried out? Is there evidence that we still need to be involved? Is there still a risk to the patient? If so, continue. This self-monitoring and self-reflection are paramount to our legal duty and autonomy. The clinician discussing the end of the treatment process needs to allow sufficient time to discuss the next steps. If outcomes have been reached, but the client still has a need, discharge can be problematic, and more time than usual may need to be allocated to discuss the impact of this.

An example of advanced reflective thinking

Anya, a speech and language therapist, was reviewing Coran, aged 19, who had been prescribed an electronic speech synthesised communication aid around two years ago. Coran has cerebral palsy, and was now at his local college of further education. He was no longer using the aid as it broke within a few months, but relied on a large ring binder, containing pictures, symbols and photographs that his mother had made up for him, to communicate. The referral requested that the therapist review his current methods of communication.

Anya, on receipt of this referral, was mindful that she did not feel qualified to assess, discuss or advise Coran and his parents on the type of aids required, so immediately referred on to a specialist communication aids centre in the area, along with a referral to the local specialist speech and language therapist, who could provide local support and back-up. She felt there was no role for her in supporting Coran, other than advising him of the onward referral.

However, having reflected on her role, and discussed it with some colleagues in peer supervision, one of whom mentioned an article she could read,[34] which discussed the therapy role with AAC users (those requiring an additional – possibly electronic – method of communication) and recommended consideration of barriers to using communication aids:
➤ the availability of specialist provision
➤ the knowledge and skill levels of practitioners
➤ the need for training for school staff
➤ the need for team working
➤ the need for someone to provide ongoing advice on technical issues, maintenance and repair
➤ the influence of attitudes and responses from those interacting with AAC users.

---

34 Baxter S, Enderby P, Evans P, *et al*. Barriers and facilitators to the use of the high-technology augmentative and alternative communication devices: a systemic review and qualitative synthesis. *IJLCD*. 2012; 47(2): 115–25.

Following this, Anya felt more confident, and used the appointment to see whether she had any role in supporting Coran at a local level when he returned with his new aid. One of her roles could be to liaise with and train college staff. She could find out more about Coran's communication network and to work on supporting him with any strategies needed to support him in daily use of the aid, depending on how those around him responded to his use of it. She might need to check that he and his family have a contact for someone who will provide ongoing advice on technical issues, maintenance and repair.

Initially, Anya did not feel she had any role in supporting Coran, but was supported in developing her thinking by listening to colleagues and reading around the subject. She took charge of her learning needs assertively, and did not passively withdraw from the situation through fear of making a mistake or not wanting to put the effort in. She thus reflected on her competence levels before, during and after the consultation. She questioned her own ability to make an impact, she asked herself who would need to be involved, what her and other's role would be, where the consultations would need to take place, when the various practitioners should be involved, and why.

It is through working reflectively that we develop our own understanding of the situation and also empathy for other's experiences and perspective. We must first understand ourselves before we can understand others. We need to see another experience in the other's own terms rather than through our own distorted interpretation. Reflection can be cathartic, as through reflection, particularly of our mistakes, we have understanding of, and maybe expression of, strong feelings. This may provoke further action.

Reflection improves our understanding of ourselves, others and professional values. Once we have mastered the ability to reflect on an experience, we become able to pause within a particular experience or situation in order to understand, reframe and change it towards a better outcome. We develop the ability to feel and respond in the unfolding moment. We develop the space to change our ideas rather than being fixed in a particular mind-set. As Williamson recommends, 'through this individual practice is continually open to challenge and improvement'.[35] The reflection will highlight learning needs, possible new ways of working, and help the clinician make changes in their practice. In this way, the clinician is open to enlightenment and empowerment.

Models of reflective practice, and approaches, may differ among different professional groups, with reflection being an individual, team, group or organisational process, conducted at any level within the organisation. As we will see in the next chapter, it is only through the process of reflection that we can seriously challenge our clinical thinking, pushing us to think in new ways

---

35 Williamson K. The best things for the best reasons. *RCSLT Bulletin*. 2000; **582**: 17–18.

that challenge the status quo and enable us to move our practice forward to face the demands set by the new NHS.

KEY POINTS

➤ Clinically, morally and professionally, we have a commitment to deliver care to the very best standard, efficiently, effectively and at the best price.

➤ We need to discuss expectations with patients, so that they are prepared – forewarned – about the limits of any treatment and their expectations are not raised unnecessarily.

➤ Users of our services will have different expectations, influenced by factors such as their own cultural and family models of healthcare, ways of managing their own health, previous use of services and perceptions of illness severity.

➤ A shift towards efficiency does not need to mean we lose the ability to connect with one another, and value things that nourish, support and nurture all of us through life, nor that we relinquish NHS values.

➤ We need to ensure that we obtain the necessary professional and clinical support structures, to ensure good access to training, clinical supervision, peer review and case discussion.

➤ The NHS has to meet a whole raft of national, political and social expectation: to provide value for money, increase patient choice, improve the patient experience, reduce inequalities, improve performance year on year and provide a platform to support public health, in addition to providing safe, effective and innovative care.

➤ Our patients may need to be brought gently into a different way of looking at their NHS, and the need for them to incorporate some level of responsibility to contribute to their own healthcare rather than simply be a passive, dependent recipient of that care.

➤ There will always be a major tension between providing the very best clinical care and the cost of that care. And practising the very best medicine at all times is impossible – the aim must always be to minimise the risk of harm. We need to ensure that our practice is client focussed and evidence based. Evidence-based practice provides us with real and solid reasons for providing the services we select.

➤ In order to clarify our thinking and decision making, and strengthen our evidence-based practice, we need to reflect constantly on our practice. It is through the process of challenging current practice that new ideas, knowledge and theory develop; the process enables us to respond to critical challenges set by the public, management or a court of law.

➤ It is through the consideration of the perspective of different people that learning occurs. We learn to gain perspective, analyse and challenge the experience from above.

➤ The application of reflective practice is apparent when we plan care for patients at a macro (strategic) and micro (local) level, in both the overall delivery of care and the care planning process applied to individual patients and clients.

➤ One of the most important principles is the support and development of thinking which challenges us personally and professionally, and requires a high level of planning, reflection and assertiveness skills.

➤ To be truly patient-centred, we need to remember that the only impact we have concerns about is the impact of our intervention(s) on the patient.

➤ Reflection improves our understanding of ourselves, and others. Once we have mastered the ability to reflect on an experience, we become able to pause within a particular experience or situation in order to understand, reframe and change it towards a better outcome. We develop the ability to feel and respond in the unfolding moment. We develop the space to change our ideas rather than being fixed in a particular mind-set.

FURTHER READING

Publications on evidence-based practice

The UK Cochrane Centre (UKCC) was established at the end of 1992 by the National Health Service Research and Development Programme and is now part of the National Institute for Health Research. It provides training and support; acts as a knowledge broker for the Cochrane Reviews; and runs a programme of methodology research and audit. It is a key link between the Collaboration, the Cochrane Reviews and the NHS. *See* www.ukcc.cochrane.org (accessed April 2013).

Bandolier: a monthly newsletter describing evidence-based thinking about healthcare and healthcare effectiveness. *See* www.medicine.ox.ac.uk/bandolier/ (accessed April 2013).

Quality Assessment in General Practice. National Primary Care Research and Development Centre. *See* www.npcrdc.man.ac.uk (accessed April 2013).

Effective Health Care bulletins: based on a systematic review and synthesis of research on the clinical effect, cost-effectiveness and acceptability of health service interventions. From 1992 to 2004 the *Effective Health Care* bulletins played a central role in the development and promotion of evidence-based practice in the NHS. Royal Society of Medicine Press. PO Box 9002, London W1A 0ZA, www.york.ac.uk (accessed April 2013).

There are many other profession-specific websites, which assist us in our quest for evidence-based practice. Currently recommended are:

➤ Medline: www.nlm.nih.gov/bsd/pmresources.html (accessed April 2013).

➤ Database of Abstracts, Abstracts of Reviews and Effects (DARE): www.crd.york.ac.uk/crdweb/ (accessed April 2013).

➤ Turning Research into Practice (TRIP): www.ncbi.nlm.nih.gov/pmc/articles/PMC1852635/ (accessed April 2013).

CHAPTER 11

Developing reflective thinking

'We don't "own" our clinical expertise: we need to think to ourselves: Is this something I can do myself, or something I can help someone else do?'[1]

In the previous chapter we began to explore some of the ways we as clinicians work reflectively to perfect our own clinical decision making. One of the difficulties in defining the competence of a healthcare worker is that competence depends on more than technical knowledge and expertise. At a deeper level still are personal attitudes, attributes and belief systems, which have an unconscious effect on our choices at the knowledge and skills level.[2] Furthermore, reflective practice both influences our future decision making and redefines our definition of competence.[3] One of the markers of developing clinical expertise is no longer being bound by rules and procedures, the technical aspects of our jobs, but allowing ourselves to look outside the box, adapt and improvise within current theory, and make personal judgements based on what we have learned: an integral part of our clinical/professional development.

One of our starting points is whether we adhere to the medical or social model of care. Here we need to consider our own value judgements, which begin to connect our own moral and ethical values to the business we are in.

A medical model is based on the premise that illness or disability is a deviation from the 'norm' – either a physical, behavioural or developmental norm. The role of the clinician is to effect a change in the individual's physical, emotional or sensory state to bring them closer to the 'norm'.

In contrast, the social model of care is based on an understanding that a client's experience of disability or impairment is placed within a broader societal context.[4] It is society's barriers that restrict the individual, not the intrinsic characteristics of their condition. Our role then is not to 'fix', but to

1 Parkin S. *RCSLT Bulletin*. 2011; **12**: 30.
2 Anderson C, van der Gaag A, editors. *Speech and Language Therapy: issues in professional practice*. Whurr Publishers Ltd; 2005. Ch. 1, p. 2.
3 Williamson K. Capable, confident and competent. *RCSLT Bulletin*. 2001; **562**: 17–18.
4 Swaine J, Finkelstein V, French S, *et al.*, editors. *Disabling Barriers: enabling environments*. Sage; 1993.

work with the individual to understand the impact of the disability and address any context-driven issues of importance to their everyday life.[5] Within this, the traditional role of 'rehabilitation' is rejected and we as the clinicians are seen as a resource, the facilitators informing not leading the process of change. The change belongs to the service user, the client/patient; the power is in the hands of the one disabled.[6] Society's role, then, is to reconfigure the disabled identity in a new, more positive and celebratory light.[7]

This chapter looks closely at the work that has been on going in the NHS and social care for the last 20 years or so, which encourages us to reflect on the core building blocks of clinical effectiveness, evidence base and risk. This builds on the conceptual framework set out in the last few chapters, when we looked at some of the newer possibilities in working collaboratively with the patient/client as an expert, and challenges the traditional, paternalistic, power base of medicine. Some of this work has been conceptualised by Malcomess and others[8] in working with a variety of client groups with chronic conditions, in particular, from adult neurology, stammering, mental health, drug and alcohol use, etc. It represents a model of thinking rather than a model of clinical care delivery, and looks at the reasons for, and delivery of, care, so its principles can be applied universally to any healthcare situation. It requires a shift of thinking based on reflection (Malcomess terms this a 'paradigm shift'), with the focus on the *impact* of the illness/disease/disorder on the person, not the diagnosis. Thus it reflects a social, not medical model of care. It offers practitioners a philosophy of practice,[9] so that instead of automatically accepting we are the best person to help those in need, we begin to examine our thought processes, and instead question *if* we are the best person to help and, if so, what is the most effective way to help?[10]

---

5   Anderson, van der Gaag, note 2 above. Keith L. *Take up Thy Bed and Walk: death, disability, and cure in classic fiction for girls*. The Women's Press; 2001.

6   Woolley M. Acquiring hearing loss: acquired oppression. In: Swaine J, Finkelstein V, French S, *et al.*, editors. *Disabling Barriers: enabling environments*. Sage; 1993.

7   Phillips MJ. Damaged goods: oral narratives of the experience of disability in American culture. *Social Science Medicine*. 1990; **30**: 849–57. Swinburn K. Journeys with aphasia: personal reflections. In: Anderson C, van der Gaag A, editors. *Speech and Language Therapy: issues in professional practice*. Whurr Publishers Ltd; 2005. Ch. 7, p. 117.

8   Malcomess K. The Care Aims model. In: Anderson C, van der Gaag A, editors. *Speech and Language Therapy: issues in professional practice*. Whurr Publishers Ltd; 2005. Ch. 4, pp. 43–71. Beirne P. Implementation of the Care Aims: challenges and opportunities. In: Anderson C, van der Gaag A, editors. *Speech and Language Therapy: issues in professional practice*. Whurr Publishers Ltd; 2005. Ch. 5, pp. 72–85. Connect, the disability network: www.connect.org (accessed April 2013). Simpson S, Sparkes C. Goal negotiation (2). Whose goal is it anyway? Part 2: Getting the process right. *Speech and Language Therapy in Practice*. 2011; Summer: 10–12. Available at: www.intandem.co.uk/ (accessed April 2013).

9   Anderson, van der Gaag, note 2 above, p. 7.

10 Malcomess, note 8 above. Beirne, note 8 above.

➤ **Who** can best help? If not me, can someone else do it better, cheaper, sooner?

➤ **Why** is the person in need of help? They may have a problem, but can we help them?

➤ **What** will best help for them? Patients may ask for antibiotics, but we know these are no help in a viral infection. We understand that a child has global learning difficulties, but there is no speedy, magic cure for this: we may best spend our time supporting the parents in understanding the diagnosis.

➤ **Where** is the best place to support them? Perhaps not in clinic but in some other agency – the drug support team, counsellors, school, parents or some other agency can deliver a programme better.

➤ **How** can they best be helped? Possibly not by medicine, but by an ongoing programme of treatment or support delivered by X, Y, Z.

At one end of the medical versus social model continuum, we see ourselves as the 'expert'; at the other, the client is the expert and we are the facilitator. Practitioners may need to accept that they might not be the one, and it might not be possible, to 'fix' the problem or the patient/client. This concept especially challenges providers of healthcare for chronic or unusual conditions, when we often become fixated with a determination to problem solve. The rapid advances in medical technology support the belief that there will be a medical solution for everything. We may have to acknowledge that this attitude brings uncertainty for the patient, who continually holds out hope for cure instead of settling into a quiet acceptance of, and adaptation to, their condition.

Client-centred care means asking a whole new set of questions, as outlined by Swinburn as she reflects on the issues facing her as a clinician working with clients with aphasia.[11]

➤ What does the person want and need to do, that is currently inaccessible to them?

➤ How much time are we likely to have as a clinical partnership?

➤ Am I clear about the options I can offer: how much, how often, the benefits, the drawbacks?

➤ Do I know what each option is targeting in terms of expected outcome?

➤ How will each option demonstrate the person's competence?

Being clinically effective involves knowing both when and how to help, as well as when to withdraw. Intervention can be harmful: consider the physical, psychological and functional effects of some of the treatments we may recommend. Medicine can pathologise, and the very nature of our work

---

11 Swinburn, note 7 above, Ch. 7, p. 123.

– investigating for and finding problems – can set up a pathology where there had been none. The social model considers that groups of people become 'problems' when defined by others as problems. The deaf community, the lesbian, gay, bisexual and transgender community, those with a disability, have all argued for autonomy and freedom from 'experts' defining what is a problem for them, deciding what is right for them. When medicine finds a deficit, it identifies an intervention. Ethically, it is not for us to define a deficit if none exists.

We do not 'own' those we care for, and as soon as we become involved we set up a cycle of dependency, where we have the power to solve the problems, and the patient thus becomes a passive recipient of our care. It is not our role to meddle in people's lives and create this dependency. It is our role to empower.

We need to move away from being 'treatment centred' and instead become 'people centred'. In order to do this, we need to focus on the clients' needs (not our need to 'mend', nor the referrer's need to solve a problem). Patients are too caught up in this approach: when they say, 'I need three times weekly therapy/antibiotics', they are describing an input not an outcome. So, one way to turn this around is get the patient to think with you about meeting the need more intelligently: 'One way to meet this need is X; another is Y.'

MANAGING THE RISK

For readers interested in the model, I refer them to the Malcomess's work on Care Aims,[12] which also offers practitioners a systematic way of recording their decisions, supporting the increasing need for accountability. Malcomess creates a framework for the building blocks of clinical reasoning, from pre-referral to post-discharge. She discusses the clinical risk to patients – physical, psychological and functional – and what may contribute to that risk, which we will look at in more detail in the next chapter. Here, I will focus more on the philosophical aspect of the model – the development of our thinking as practitioners.

As NHS professionals, we have a statutory duty of care, based on the principles outlined in legislation, to patients we accept for treatment. It is for us, as autonomous professionals, to interpret clinical need, and for us to accept the referral if the patient is both at high risk *and* we have something to offer them. We have the skills to define what is a reasonable judgement, based on the care given by anyone of the same seniority or professional standing. As we have noted previously, our statutory duty is to do the most good and the least harm for the most number of people, and as part of that duty we have to accept that risk assessment skills are central. We are personally and professionally

---

12 Malcomess, note 8 above.

accountable for our decisions, and must be in a position to explain our clinical reasoning to anyone who may ask, We cannot hide behind our employer; we cannot hide behind protocols or say we were not given enough time/equipment to complete the job. Within the NHS we have a duty to assess only, not treat: people cannot demand we treat if we do not feel it is appropriate.

Here we look at how to apply robust clinical thinking, and how to hold the boundary, at all stages of the client journey.

1   Triage – can we help here?

Many teams now have triage processes in place, to ensure that referrals received are screened, and consideration given to how the team can best help the patient. To help in this process, and to help clinicians begin to widen their thinking and hold a boundary, this team would benefit from giving careful consideration to the following.

➤ The appropriateness of the referral: are we best able to help here? Is this our responsibility?

➤ The likelihood that the referral will be beneficial to the client.

➤ The adequacy of the client's consent for the referral: if in any doubt, seek for information from the referrer before consenting to accepting the referral.

2   Accepting the referral – and how do we plan to intervene?

Once we agree to take on a patient, especially a patient or client with a chronic, ongoing condition, we constantly have to ask ourselves the following questions.

➤ What is my duty here?

➤ How do I know I am discharging my duty effectively?

➤ How do I know when I no longer have a duty?

➤ Who else has a duty to this person? Can I help them discharge their duty? How?

➤ Is the client/family aware of my involvement and my duty at each stage?

➤ Have I clarified how I am going to deliver the care? And how any changes to the agreement will be managed? If treatment has been limited in some way – say to a prescribed number of sessions – consider the best ways to communicate this. Perhaps: 'We have eight sessions to work, together with this time together. At session 6 we will consider together whether we have met these goals and if we feel we need more time/an extension.'

➤ It is always good to make treatments time-limited? Continue seeing anyone while you are making an impact, while they show progress. If you keep someone on beyond this boundary, consider what your motives are for continuing. Are you hoping to care/cure/save/heal? Is this our role? We cannot save anyone.

This is all about working efficiently and managing risk. This approach tells us there are some fundamental assumptions we need to take into account when managing risk.

1   We must target vulnerable populations and help them to manage their own risk, where possible. Prevention is much better than cure, and helping the population manage their own risk is by far the most effective way of improving their health and well-being. Hence the huge rise in expert patient programmes, training packages to support people with managing the risk.

2   Healthcare is not a right. We must provide care for the biggest number of people, but we do need to prioritise those who need the focus of our care. Once we have accepted a referral, we have a duty to assess, and, if we are not taking the patient on, to hand back responsibility to the referrer swiftly, clearly and effectively: we are then clear we are not taking on a duty of care, nor are we the right person to manage the risk.

3   We must support other professionals to manage risk by giving them the skills in identification and risk management.

4   Whose risk is it? We are all safer managing our own risk. It is clearly better for a child who chokes on liquids or who has a peanut allergy to understand how to control and manage that risk as they grow up, instead of depending on parental/outside 'expert' help to manage the problem indefinitely. The risk is at a manageable level for them to deal with themselves.

In order to help us identify whether we need to take on a duty of care, we need to identify where our patients fit. Consider the following clinical scenarios.

➤ The child with cerebral palsy, whose speech, especially when tired, is difficult to understand. She has a communication aid which is rarely used, so is never charged up.

➤ The teenager with cystic fibrosis, who does not always take his medication and refuses to 'do' the exercises prescribed.

➤ The depressed adult, who attends therapy but does not comply with the homework given.

➤ The single parent who finds it hard to mix, has little spare money and rarely takes her child to pre-school appointments.

➤ The working adult who has frequent upper respiratory tract infections and 'needs' antibiotics in order to function in his busy working schedule.

➤ The elderly diabetic who is a frequent surgery attender as, for various reasons, he finds it hard to comply with the prescribed diet.

You will be able to think of your own example. Who is best placed to help these clients/patients? Yes, they need support, but at what level of intervention? Who is managing the risk? Clearly, the patients have been given the risk back to self-manage, and they are not following the advice given. But do they need more appointments to tell them this? Where could they best get the support they need? Do they need support at the self-help/public health level? At a universal level of care, which may be at school, the GP, the pharmacist, the health visitor? They may benefit from targeted care – some community support from Sure Start, Citizens Advice, a volunteer agency.

We clinicians, providing a specialist service, need to focus our support on those we can best help – the newly diagnosed, who we can assess, diagnose, advise and train, if needed. We may need to refer on to specialist regional or national services, or to a specialist diagnostic service provided for unusual or rare diagnoses. We need to be assertive about our ability to manage the patient's risk, and although risk can change and therefore may need to be reviewed regularly, it is much better to manage the risk as close to the client as possible, so that they learn to manage their own risk and use the health service only when they can no longer do so. We need to be assertive about saying to our patients: 'This is something you can manage yourself now. Come back to us if new and specific concerns arise.'

The better services being commissioned are now done so by basing funding on outcomes. The focus is not on time (the number of sessions to be given), but on an outcome. The integrated services provided by health and social care to support those living in the community are working to support the client to manage themselves. If the patient manages their own risk, they are building their own competence and capacity to manage, and this in turn reduces their level of dependency and empowers them.

So, our role as NHS clinicians is to assess, diagnose and treat the high-risk, high-clinical-need patients: but only if we can help. It is also to promote health, identify and prevent harm, and signpost access to the most appropriate service as speedily as possible. If we do our job properly, and focus on *outcomes*, we will be able to think a little more clearly about who would best help this patient, when and how. Do they need reassurance? Support or education? Do we need to help other people to do their job effectively? How can we help people to learn the skills to manage their condition? If we think that the risk can be managed more effectively by a change in attitudes or environment (as in the above clinical examples), it is not clinical intervention that is required, but educative change, applied at a public health/educational level. Specialist services, at primary and secondary care level, become involved only if change cannot be achieved at the universal level. In order to justify continuing to work with the patient, a measure of clinical outcome is required. The judgement is based on a predication of change, so it must relate to our evidence base. Each plan of work/intervention with our patient represents some degree of predicted effectiveness, where we focus on the *impact*, not the presenting problem. So we continually ask: are we being effective? Are we making a difference? Are we making an impact? Can we justify our reasoning? Can we predict change? If not, we must discharge the patient and duty of care to someone who is able to make an impact.

While we hold a duty of care, we are clinically responsible for that patient. This is, quite rightly, a big responsibility, and we do need to be able to justify why we feel we are the right people to hold that responsibility.

3 Treatment: working collaboratively

We have identified that, historically, our decision making has often been clinically driven, based on the condition not the presenting circumstances. To help us move on from this, we need to work collaboratively with the client/patient to unpick the presenting problem. Here are some questions that may help the unpicking so that we can ascertain the real, and the perceived, impact of the problem, and also find out more about what the client's underlying knowledge/assumptions are of his or her disease/problem.

Unpicking the story

Why?
Why have you come to see me today?
Why are you coming for help *now*?
Why is this a problem for you?

What?
What have you done so far? Did it help?
What do others in your life – your family and friends – think about this?
What is it that you would like to be able to do/achieve that you feel unable to do now?
What do you think this might mean for you?
What do you think would happen without my help?

How?
How are you coping at the moment?
How do you feel about this?
Are there any situations in which this is not a problem for you? How come?
Are you currently receiving help for this?
How does this affect your life?
How has this changed your activity/life?
How much do you understand about this diagnosis?
How do you think I can help you?

Who?

In your family, who is most affected?

Who do you think can help you with this? Is it me? Who else has/can help?

What have you been told that a health visitor/district nurse/therapist/doctor does with this problem? What are your expectations?

Use this type of questioning to open up the problem, and to show the patient/client that – in many instances of minor illnesses – there may indeed be a difficulty, but that that difficulty may not necessarily be solved with drugs/therapy/input from the healthcare team. There are many difficulties that just are, and no magic solution can be found to manage them. Not only that, but sometimes life is no different before, during or after the illness, but the patient/client has focussed on the illness as the main problem in their lives.

In the West, we live in a consumerist society: we have come to expect that we can pay for our way out of difficulties, and we expect those around us to collude with that. We may need to consider how our lives would be different if we woke up and our difficulties/problems had disappeared. The questions guide, not prescribe: they are used to help you, and the patient, think. The aim is to develop a shared understanding of the problem and to set goals to resolve it with the patient and their carers.

If we ask the above questions actively and with empathy, we are asking, not promising; we are focussing on outcomes, not input. We focus on enabling the client to think, and facilitate mutual understanding, and we maintain clear boundaries around our responsibilities. We are solution focussed, not problem focused, and this is where the advanced clinical thinking and ability to assertively set boundaries begins.

When negotiating goals with the client, Simpson and Sparkes recommend that you focus on the following at different stages of the process,[13] here annotated.

1 Develop a list of the client's strengths, needs, wants and issues. This may be an individual list, if working solely with the client, or a collective list, if working as part of a multidisciplinary team.

2 Explain the process of goal negotiation: this enhances the client's knowledge of the service and how that service is delivered in addition to its specific remit and boundaries. This is integral to managing both client and professional expectations.

3 Explore the lifestyle issues, wants and aspirations, so that more client-centred goals can be elicited.

---

13 Simpson, Sparkes, note 8 above.

4 Develop the prerequisites for goal negotiation. The client's capacity to negotiate meaningful goals will depend on their:
  a personality
  b life experience
  c degree of emotional stability
  d level of cognitive understanding
  e capacity for mature reflection, self-understanding and decision making.
  Through this you will be able to establish the client's potential to change.
5 Goal elicitation: develop frameworks including prioritisation, rating scales and steps, option appraisal. Use information collected by each discipline if working in a team.

Simpson and Sparkes also recommend regular, ongoing goal negotiation meetings, to agree and review all long-term/discharge goals, short-terms goals, and plans of action, and to help maintain focus and review effectiveness of interventions. At the final goal negotiation meeting you review all the goals and the overall intervention package, evaluate from the client's perspective, discuss endings and identify any future goal areas. Throughout, we should be using adult-centred communication, applying empowering self-educating messages, and not endlessly delivering professional opinions, which demeans those we assist and makes them unequal in the relationship.[14]

Motivational interviewing[15]

If we return to the above clinical scenarios where the patients have not taken responsibility for following advice given, there are ways to help them see more clearly where the lines of responsibility lie. Two possible methods are outlined here. The first, motivational interviewing (MI), is based on an intervention commonly used by clinicians working with alcohol awareness. The Screening and Prevention Programme for Sensible Drinking[16] (SIPS) alcohol screening

14 Ferguson A, Armstrong E. Reflections on speech – language therapists talk; implications for clinical practice and education. *International Journal of Language & Communication Disorders*. 2004; **39**(4): 469–507.

15 Miller WR, Rollnick S. *Motivational Interviewing: preparing people to change addictive behaviour*. The Guilford Press; 1991.

16 Coulton S, Perryman K, Cassidy P, *et al.* Screening and brief interventions for hazardous alcohol use in accident and emergency departments: a randomised controlled trial protocol. *BMC Health Services Research*. 2009; **9**: 114. Kaner E, Bland M, Cassidy P, *et al.* Screening and brief interventions for hazardous and harmful alcohol use in primary care: a cluster randomised controlled trial protocol. *BMC Public Health*. 2009; **9**: 287. Newbury-Birch D, Bland M, Cassidy P, *et al.* Screening and brief interventions for hazardous and harmful alcohol use in probation services: a cluster randomised controlled trial protocol. *BMC Public Health*. 2009; **9**: 418.

and brief intervention (ASBI) research programme was funded by the UK Department of Health in 2006 as part of the national Alcohol Harm Reduction Strategy for England. The programme comprised three cluster randomised controlled trials of different methods of screening and brief intervention across three settings: primary healthcare, emergency departments and probation services. The main aims of the programme were to evaluate the effectiveness and cost effectiveness of different methods of screening and brief interventions for alcohol misuse and to assess the feasibility of, and factors promoting or inhibiting, implementation in the typical practice setting.

MI has been used by psychologists for some time in supporting people with managing change and helping them to accept and understand the ambivalence that gets in the way of behavioural change. MI is used in addictions treatment and other clinical contexts, and has applications in medical, public health and criminal justice settings. It is used successfully with groups, couples and adolescents. In essence, it empowers people to become ready, willing and able to make changes that improve the quality of their lives.

We can use MI in supporting patients to manage change. Here, the author has adapted the MI technique for use in a therapeutic setting, and the example given is used now in a paediatric integrated therapy service, for physio, occupational, and speech and language therapists to use with parents and their children:

➤ to identify both the skill level of the child and the parent and establish whether they want to work on the needs
➤ when there is a discrepancy between the motivation of the child and their helpers
➤ for older children/teenagers
➤ if the child or parent is non-compliant or very anxious
➤ if the interview is proving to be challenging
➤ in the context of helping parents come to terms with their child's discharge, if discharge is proving challenging or if the child has significant and ongoing needs that the service can no longer address.

The approach demands a high level of clinical skill and experience, as it can challenge traditional thinking, especially for parents who have come to expect 'wrap around care', a cradle-to-grave service. Whoever uses the approach needs to be assertive, needs to use excellent communication skills, and so must discuss the child's needs with honesty, care and compassion.

The checklist is used to unpick underlying concerns, and to identify the positives and negatives about making the change. For change to occur, there needs to be more positives than negatives about making the change. If there are more negatives, it is unlikely that the goal will be achieved and this should be discussed.

An example of a motivational interviewing scale

Identify the problem. Ask:

What is your *biggest* concern? Ask this question of all interested parties: the patient, or child, or parent, for example.

What is the current impact? 'She wants to be able to ...'

What has been done so far? Has this helped? How are things different now?

Identify the motivation, skills, confidence
Use the scoring sheet either at assessment or at review to identify both the skill level of the child and how much they want to work on it.

Use a scale of 1 = not good, 10 = very good.

Problem	Skill	Motivation	Confidence
Therapist	/10	/10	/10
School	/10	/10	/10
Parent	/10	/10	/10

Skill: How *well* does the child currently perform this activity?

Motivation: How much do you want to do it?

Confidence: How *confident* are you that you can achieve this?

You might find it helpful to unpick these responses by asking:

Why have you have given yourself this number?

Why did you not give yourself a lower number?

A higher number?

Ask the patient to identify the good things about making a change and also the negative aspects. Remember that for change to occur there must be more positives than negatives. If there are more negatives, it is unlikely that the goal will be achieved and this should be discussed. If the parent/child is using a lot of 'change talk' (e.g. 'I am going to do X'), this is a good sign that change will occur. For change to occur, you need to have three more positives than negatives. Examples are shown below.

Positive/negative

'Mum and Dad won't go on at me.'/'Less time for Xbox if doing exercises.'

In order to change habits permanently, the patient has to be motivated to change, and this usually happens when there are more *positive* reasons to change than *negative*.

If the patient is demotivated, and unwilling to work on changing their behaviour, very often the parent, partner or carer cannot understand why the therapist/doctor/nurse cannot offer any treatment. The old adage 'you can lead a horse to water but you can't make it drink' comes to mind. No one but the patient/client themselves can effect a change, however much the parent/carer/partner wants them to change. The model below, developed by change management experts, may help explain.

Health psychology

Spiral of change (Transtheoretical model)[17]

Pre-contemplation

'Do I have a problem? If I have, I don't want to do anything about it.'

Contemplation

'I have a problem and I may want to do something about it one day.'

Preparation

'I have a problem and I want to do something about it – soon.'

Action

'I want, and am getting, some help now. I am practising daily.'

Or

'I am aware of my problem and struggle with it.'

Maintenance

'I've learnt how to help myself and will practise whenever I walk to the bus.'

Or

'I am aware of my problem and it doesn't cause me any difficulty.'

---

17 DiClemente CC, Prochaska JO. Toward a comprehensive, transtheoretical model of change: stages of change and addictive behaviors. In: Miller WR, Heather N, editors. *Treating Addictive Behaviors*. 2nd ed. Plenum Press; 1998. pp. 3–24.

> **Integration**
>
> 'I can do this most of the time in everyday life'
>
> Or
>
> 'I may still have difficulty, but is no longer a problem for me.'

The patient must be wanting help, at an 'action' level, before any therapy is effective. For more information about using the approach in treatment, *see* Chapter 12, Putting it into practice.

4   When and how to end treatment: discharge and empowerment

This is the point we are all working towards. Our overall aim is to plan care that can empower the patient/client and their carer and support them towards independence and managing conditions for themselves. We want to discourage any unnecessary dependency on services. To help us do this, we need to forget the 'problems' that present, and instead focus on the main presenting difficulties and their current impact. As part of coming to this more developed thinking, we may need to unpick what the patient or their carer wants to be different and think how best this can be achieved. Will it happen anyway without your help? To recap: keep asking yourself *why* you are helping. If you cannot answer that, you should not be helping. Think about *whose* need is being met – the child's, the parents', school's, the service's or yours? Your focus must be the patient or client, it is they we have responsibility for, not their family/school/neighbours/friends.

Before we consider discharging the patient, we must know our own service inside out. Different settings have different ways of working. Consider how time is framed and boundaries are determined. Does your service offer a standard time-limited contract? Or are more discrete, flexible packages on offer? Are admission and discharge graded? Can the work be adjusted in accordance with the client's readiness for change and the focus of therapy? Is your service a single disciplinary one or multidisciplinary and, if multiple, what is the impact of discharging from part of the service offered?

In most NHS service, people are thrilled to be discharged: it is a welcome confirmation that there is no longer any problem. However, some services have a problem with a dependency culture, for example, if:

➤ the patient has a chronic illness, or a long-term difficulty
➤ the patient has had high dependency needs – perhaps long-term input as an outpatient or, if a child, intensive input from, for example, an opportunity playgroup or special school.

If this patient/child has had 'wrap around care' from previous services, some dependency has been set up and there may be an expectation that a high level of input will continue. Sometimes the discharging team does not check whether anything can be done before referring on to a new service. They may do this, as, unassertively, they may wish to avoid confrontation and discussion with the patient about the reality of the situation, or they may simply not know.

In the West, we are somewhat handicapped by a level of richness that enables us to want, demand and expect more. We no longer accept mediocrity or substandard behaviour, and demand the highest level of care from all public services. Parents, rightly, are especially demanding of the very best level of care for their children. In paediatric work, teams are often asked to see children who have global developmental difficulties, but no specific difficulty that is out of line with their general developmental age. These are children who certainly do have noticeable problems with their speech/language/walking/co-ordination/ social skills, but these difficulties may be developmentally appropriate. Contrary to parental expectation and understanding, developmental disorders are not diseases that one either has or does not; they are behaviourally defined dimensional traits along a continuum, with fuzzy edges and a wide range of severity.[18]

It is hard to explain to their carers – the referrer, school, parents – that we have no magic wand to wave, the child's presentation is in line with their developmental age, and no amount of intervention/surgery/medication/ therapy/exercise/labelling will change this presentation. Parents often seek, or push for, a diagnosis, a label. If children are categorised into a particular group, there is a danger that misleading expectations may be set up which mask or underplay the child's real difficulties. Therefore, it is often better in this scenario to profile strengths and weaknesses rather than to make diagnostic classifications. Clinicians need to hold a firm boundary and not let themselves be swayed by parental demands.

With developmental disorders, the schools/parents/referrers are often stuck in the frame of 'there is a difficulty', rather than 'there is a difficulty and can I do something about it'. It is these children who are re-referred repeatedly, and help is often sought in the independent sector, where doctors and therapists are possibly willing to raise parental hopes and expectations. Similarly, many people seek out plastic surgery to enhance their body shape or image, thinking that this will make a difference. They may be shocked when the breast implant has made them feel better, but now their buttocks look droopy. And what about the batwing arms? A materialistic approach and capitalism can help feed the idea that more is best, money can and will solve the problem.

Clinicians can help to unpick and prevent this way of thinking if they:

---

18 Farmer M, Oliver A. Assessment of pragmatic difficulties and socio-emotional adjustment in practice. *IJLCD*. 2005; **40**(4): 403–29.

> ➤ are entirely honest about expectations: is this a cure or a therapy?
> ➤ identify the expected outcome at the beginning of care
> ➤ agree how change will be evaluated
> ➤ engage the client/patient in all ongoing discussions about their care
> ➤ review their decision on a regular basis by evaluating the outcome against any baseline measurements.

If you are honest about the expected outcome, then the client is clear about progress made and is prepared for discharge. If you have not worked in this systematic way, and the patient has been on the books for a long time without evident progress but a lot of ongoing 'support', you may need to 'signpost' discharge in advance. Giving service users 'contracts of care' helps to support this process – here a discussion on their expectations will be held and the clinician has a chance to explain what absolutely can and cannot be done. The clinician must make it clear that the problem may always feature, but that it is hoped that strategies can be developed which will help to support people in coming to terms with, and managing, themselves and their condition in the long term. Following this clarification, when the time comes to discharge, they can be reminded about the initial discussion on the clinician's role, any further support they may need and who is best placed to give that support.
The following phrases may help.[19]

> ➤ 'I'm wondering what I can offer and how you feel I can help given the work we have already done on …'
> ➤ 'Try this exercise/tablets/ diet and come back if there are any problems.'
> ➤ 'We will discharge, but do come back to us if your needs or circumstances change.'
> ➤ 'You have made good progress and your skills/body/abilities are now within the normal range.'
> ➤ 'You have made good progress and although your skills are still a bit delayed, they are developing following a normal pattern and should continue to do so.'
> ➤ 'Can you explain why you want my continued involvement?'
> ➤ 'Although you still has difficulties in …, the advice that has already been given is still relevant and no new advice can be given at this time.'
> ➤ 'As your child is not concerned about …, any therapy is unlikely to be successful.'
> ➤ 'If the difficulty doesn't resolve in the next year, please ring our advice line to find out whether we need to see you again.'

---

19 With thanks to the Care Planning champions, Integrated Paediatric Therapy Services, Somerset Partnership NHS Trust.

➤ 'I'm wondering what I can offer and how you feel I can help given the work we have already done.'
➤ 'We have addressed all X's current needs and it is time to transfer their care back to the school/GP.'
➤ 'Give this a go and come back if there are any problems.'
➤ 'Phone or refer back to us if your needs or circumstances change.'
➤ 'I could review you again in six months, but I don't think I would be able to add anything to what I have already said.'

A clear, assertive and immediate discharge is preferable, without prevarication. However, it can be helpful to delay a discharge by offering to discharge after a set time (perhaps three to six months), to give the patient/client time to consider it. They can be asked to contact you before the agreed period is over if they have concerns; otherwise you will discharge. And if they do contact you during that time, you may need to revisit the discussion around the following.

➤ How do you think I can help?
➤ What can I offer you that is new?
➤ Has something changed?

If things remain as they were, the patient will begin to understand, eventually, that you have nothing new to offer and work with them stops.

KEY POINTS
➤ Personal attitudes, attributes and belief systems all have an unconscious effect on our choices at the knowledge and skills level of our competence.
➤ One of the markers of developing clinical expertise is no longer being bound by the technical aspects of our jobs, but allowing ourselves to look outside the box, adapt and improvise within current theory, and make personal judgements based on what we have learned.
➤ One of our starting points is whether we adhere to the medical or social model of care. Here we need to consider our own value judgements, which begin to connect our own moral and ethical values to the business we are in.
➤ The social model of care is based on an understanding that a client's experience of disability or impairment is placed within a broader societal context. Our role is thus to work with the individual to address the context-driven issues of importance to their everyday life.
➤ Working collaboratively with the patient challenges the traditional, paternalistic power base of medicine. It represents a model of thinking rather than a model of clinical care delivery, with the focus on the impact of the illness/disease/disorder on the person, not the diagnosis. Ethically,

it is not for us to define a deficit if it does not exist, or is not defined by the patient/client. If there is no impact, we must withdraw. Conversely, people cannot demand we treat if we do not feel it is clinically appropriate.

➤ Are we clear, within this, about the options we offer: how much, how often, the benefits, the drawbacks? Can we demonstrate how each option aids the person's competence?

➤ At one end of the medical versus social model continuum, we see ourselves as the 'expert'; at the other, the client is the expert and we are the facilitator.

➤ Clinicians may need to accept that they might not be the one, and it might not be possible, to 'fix' the problem or the patient. This concept especially challenges providers of healthcare for chronic or unusual conditions, when we often get fixated with a determination to problem solve. We may have to acknowledge uncertainty.

➤ Being clinically effective involves knowing both when and how to help, as well as when to withdraw. Intervention can be harmful. It can pathologise and create dependency.

➤ We are personally and professionally accountable for our decisions, and must be in a position to explain our clinical reasoning to anyone who may ask – we cannot hide behind our employer.

➤ Clinical teams need to be assertive about, and perfect their boundary keeping at triage, accepting the referral (do and how do we plan to intervene?), advice and treatment (who is best placed to treat?), and discharge. Different settings have different ways of working. Consider how time is framed and boundaries are determined.

➤ Healthcare is not a right. We must provide care for the biggest number of people, but we do need to prioritise those who need the focus of our care. We must support our patients and other professionals to manage risk by giving them the skills in identification and risk management.

➤ In order to justify continuing to work with a patient, clinical outcome is required. The judgement is based on a predication of change, so it must relate to our evidence base. We continually need to ask: are we being effective? Are we making a difference? Are we making an impact? Can we justify our reasoning? Can we predict change? If not, we must discharge the patient and duty of care to someone who is able to make an impact.

➤ We need to work collaboratively with the client/patient to unpick the presenting problem, so we can ascertain the real, and the perceived, impact of the problem, and also find out more about the patient's underlying knowledge/assumptions of their disease. We do this through judicious questioning. The aim is to develop a shared understanding of the problem and set goals to resolve it with the patient and their carers.

➤ Throughout, we should use adult-centred communication, applying empowering self-educating messages, and not endlessly deliver professional opinions, which demeans patients and makes them unequal in the relationship.

➤ Motivational interviewing (MI), and the Transtheoretical model can be used in supporting people with managing change and helping them to overcome the ambivalence which gets in the way of behavioural change.

➤ In the West, we are somewhat handicapped by a level of richness that enables us to want, demand and expect more. We no longer accept mediocrity or substandard behaviour, and demand the highest level of care from all public services. This is why it is hard to explain to people that there may be nothing else we can do. Capitalism can help feed the idea that more is best, money can and will solve the problem. Clinicians can help to unpick and prevent this way of thinking if they use contracts of care, are honest about expectations, identify expected outcomes, agree how change will be evaluated and signpost discharge.

FURTHER READING

Burbank P, Riebe D, editors. *Promoting Exercise and Behavior Change in Older Adults: interventions with the transtheoretical model.* Springer Publishing Co. Inc.; 2001.

Klar Y, Fisher JD, Chinsky JM, *et al.*, editors. *Self Change: social psychological and clinical perspectives.* Springer Publishing Co. Inc.; 1992.

CHAPTER 12

Putting it into practice for the patient

In the next three chapters, we look at how to develop our interpersonal communication skills to support our clinical work. For our purposes, the concern is to develop our clinical thinking so we begin to:

➤ work in a client-centred way, using the social, not medical model
➤ reflect on our thinking continually while working, pause and reflect on how effective we are being
➤ develop assertiveness skills so we challenge the status quo where appropriate; and challenge our colleagues, managers and the government to think differently
➤ challenge ourselves to work more deeply, confidently and assertively with clients, moving out of our usual comfort zone, exploring unchartered waters that may provoke uncomfortable feelings.

We begin by focusing on using these skills to support the client with changing – both their sense of self and their skills. We look here at two main approaches: person-centred and behaviourist approaches. For our purposes, these are not mutually exclusive; both may be used at different stages of the patient journey to help them move on. Getting people to trust and confide in us is a real skill, and one that as clinicians we need to develop. We need to encourage open, honest and assertive communication from our patients/clients, so that we can get to the/their truth. As healthcare workers, we need to develop advanced, and excellent, interpersonal communication skills. Often called 'first line counselling skills', these are demanded of us in every aspect of our work with people, from assessment through to discharge, as they come to terms with their illness/disability and learn the skills to cope with managing it. We need to understand both their expectations and their perspective on both their condition and the service we offer.[1] Only then can we move forward into a

---

1 Glogowska M. Understanding expectations. In: Anderson C, Van der Gagg A, editors. *Speech and Language Therapy: issues in professional practice*. Whurr Publishers Ltd; 2005. Ch. 3, pp. 27–42.

care partnership of shared decision making.[2] The first section in this chapter looks at some of the ways we can encourage our clients to open up to us, and tell us their stories.

In the second part of the chapter, we look at the best ways of helping people change their own behaviour (including developing assertiveness skills), looking at some strategies we have been told teach behavioural change and some others which may be more effective. We look at some of the skills we need to develop in order to help our patients change both their behaviour and the way they think about themselves, and how to motivate and support them with making changes. Within this we examine our need to be courageous in challenging agendas that are set for us by government and management. Our personal development and professional accountability demand that we listen, but always question, and apply any recommendations with due intelligence, confidence, assertiveness and consideration for what is best for our patients/clients.

SUPPORTING PEOPLE TO TALK

In conversation, it is said there are two components beyond the verbal/non-verbal model we have already looked at. Kagan defines two components: transaction, which is concerned with the exchange of information and ideas, and interaction, which is about the process of relationship building.[3] The transaction is the more obvious, overt, verbal element; the interaction is the hidden, covert element. Both reflect the range of skill brought to an encounter in support of the patient learning to change. Part of the clinical role is to give information, explain and guide. Other roles are to facilitate, support, model and give feedback. Throughout the process of supporting our patients to see things differently, to learn and change, we need to hold awareness of these overt and covert methods of communicating, and reflect consistently on our communication styles and delivery methods.

Getting people to open up and confide in us is a real skill, and one that as clinicians we need to develop. If the patient or client has a story they need to tell, and you need to hear, they need to be able to trust that we will 'hold' the information safely and support them without judgement. Good listening, as we saw in the first section of the book, is a learned skill, and one which we need to develop. We need to encourage open, honest and assertive communication from our patients/clients, so that we can get to the/their truth. Once we have the truth we can work honestly with people to support them in the best way

---

2 Charles C, Whelan T, Gafni A. What do we mean by partnership in making decisions about treatment? *BMJ*. 1999; **319**: 780–2.
3 Kagan A. Revealing the competence of aphasic adults through conversation: a challenge to health professionals. *Topics in Stroke Rehabilitation*. 1995; **2**: 15–28.

possible with whatever it is they present with. As healthcare workers, we need to develop advanced, and excellent, interpersonal communication skills. Here we look at some of the ways we can encourage our clients to open up to us, and tell us their story. Counsellors and therapists spend a long time on learning the skills of building up trust, supporting without invading people's sense of self, and allowing other people their feelings without imposing their own on them. Here we look at some of the key, first line counselling skills they use.

Allow time to build up trust

It does take time to build up trust, and many clinicians no longer have the luxury of time. However, if in your job it is crucial to understand your client's behaviour fully, perhaps in supporting them through any number of personal or medical crises, it is really important to allow time to develop your relationship. Through the quality of this relationship a safe space will be created, and people are more likely to tell the truth about themselves without fear of being judged.

Telling the truth

We need to be completely truthful with people if we want the truth back. So caution people before you answer their questions: pre-warn them that you will be honest in your response and ask them to be mindful of their motives in asking. People need to be prepared to hear the truth.

Reflecting

We have previously discussed the importance of a level playing field, and removing or acknowledging any power imbalances in equal and honest communication. One way to help support this is by summarising what you have heard and understood. Here you are not talking from a point of authority, as you are reflecting back what you have heard: 'It seems you are telling me X ...' You are acting as a prompt. It is the client's story.

Privacy

You will need absolute privacy, a space and a time when there is time to explore the feelings. It is crucial the moment is one to one and uninterrupted: people behave quite differently and more honestly when they are alone.

Trust

People have to trust that you will not judge or question their truth. Be open to what is said, even if privately you question the rationality of it. Build up a reputation of being trustworthy. Never share confidences outside the framework you have set yourself, unless explicit permission is given. Pre-warn the client when you first meet and agree the terms of your work together. Within this, you may need to be explicit about any levels of risk: any risk to the client or others may need to be reported elsewhere, with or without their permission. Use your signed consent and safeguarding agreements to discuss this.

Allow repetition

When a person presents with a traumatic or distressing life event, they will need support in the telling and re-telling of their story. This helps them to integrate any new narrative into their lives, and to understand the new person they have become.

Allow feelings

Learn to manage your responses when people are vulnerable. Allow tears, anger – the whole range of responses. Hold your own feelings in check: this is not your space, but your patient's. Maintain a calm demeanour. This allows the person you are speaking with to understand and accept their whole range of human emotions, without fearing them or feeling humiliated or shameful about having them. Learn about your own feelings and responses so that you will be aware when your buttons are being pressed. Are you looking critical? Suspicious? Make it easy for the person to talk to you as a reliable and secure ally.

Focus on non-verbals

Be alert to the non-verbal clues you, and your patient, are giving. Watch out for unusual or defensive patterns of eye contact, posture, tone of voice, speech patterns, use of gesture. Develop an intuitive awareness to patterns of language or behaviour that suggest manipulation, lies or self-denial.

The right not to communicate

Allow people the space not to talk. We all have the right to remain silent: when it is unsafe to disclose we may feel unhappy, vulnerable and exposed. It may be more important quietly to accept the unsaid.

Recently, work has been undertaken by researchers[4] in an attempt to create a competence measure for person-centred and experiential therapists working with clients, which includes 'process subscales', adapted here. These may be seen as advanced communication processes, not all of which are requisite skills

---

4 Freire E, Elliot R, Westwell G. The person centred and experiential psychotherapy scale (PCEPS) in measuring the unmeasurable. *Therapy Today.* 2012; **23**(4): 22. Available at: www.therapytoday.net (accessed April 2013).

for clinicians other than psychological therapists, but they are useful to consider, for those wishing to further their interpersonal communication skills.

➤ **Client frame of reference:** how much do our responses convey an understanding of the client's experience, and to what extent are we following the client's track?

➤ **Core meaning:** how well do our responses reflect the essence of what our client is communicating?

➤ **Client flow:** how well are we responsively attuned, moment by moment?

➤ **Warmth:** how well does our tone of voice convey warmth?

➤ **Clarity of language:** do we communicate simply and clearly to the client?

➤ **Content directedness:** are we unnecessarily 'directing' the client, rather than following their lead?

➤ **Accepting presence:** are we accepting the material given to us unconditionally, without judgement?

➤ **Genuineness:** are our responses natural and genuine?

➤ **Psychological holding:** 'holding' the client, metaphorically, when they are experiencing painful, scary or overwhelming experiences – staying with the moment, staying with their pain.

➤ **Dominant or overpowering presence:** to what extent does the therapist project a sense of dominance or authority?

➤ **Collaboration:** how much does the therapist appropriately and skilfully facilitate client/therapist mutual involvement in the goals and tasks of therapy?

➤ **Emotion focus:** how much does the therapist work to help the client focus on and articulate their emotional experiences?

➤ **Client self-development:** how much does the therapist work to facilitate new awareness, growth, self-determination and empowerment in the client?

➤ **Emotion regulation sensitivity:** how much does the therapist work to support the client actively in productive self-exploration?

If we are going to support those we have some kind of therapeutic relationship with, these are the kinds of skills we need to develop, so that we can get the very best out of, and support, our clients with change. Part of the therapeutic role is to encourage people to see themselves in relation to their problem, instead of simply having the problem. This leads naturally to a more positive approach, to externalising rather than internalising and personalising the problem. Hence our use of who/why/what/where/when in questioning: the unpicking of a problem to identify the barriers to the patient's functioning.

Outside this therapeutic role, part of our job may be to advise, to prescribe. It needs to be remembered that of course we are not always working with the aim to encourage people to talk with us, sometimes we do need a more practical gain: Swinburn has set out some of these ideas.[5] We may talk to our client to get specific information, to find out what they want to know, to support them their decision making. We may need to check that people have understood: signpost them to different sources of information. People may have different information and motivation needs at different stages:[6] they may seek information to help them cope, in order to meet their basic needs. They may seek information to help them feel safe and secure. They may seek enlightenment or empowerment.

In this next section we look at some of the more cognitive-behavioural approaches to managing change.

CHANGING BEHAVIOUR

We now know that if we want to help people change their behaviour and the way they think about themselves, including becoming more assertive, we need to motivate and support them with making changes. The changes will not just happen by themselves, and certainly not if we simply prescribe them. People have to 'own' the changes; they have to be in charge of them. For long-term change to occur, different behaviours need to be self-initiated, maintained and within the person's own control. In order for this to happen, we need to focus on the person, not ourselves, and support and empower them. In short, we need to manage the situation assertively, keeping focussed and separate; keeping our own needs and desires for change out of the picture.

In addition, part of being assertive is to be courageous in challenging agendas that are set for us by others. Our work in healthcare is impacted by government and management agendas, and we may not always agree with some of the recommendations made. Professionally, we have a responsibility to our patients and our professions, and as such we may not agree with all of the mandates issued to us. If professionally we do not feel comfortable with any imposed agenda, we can challenge it, provided we can give good, evidence-based reasoning why it will not suit our patients. Our personal development and professional accountability demands that we listen, question and apply any recommendations with due intelligence, confidence, assertiveness and consideration for what is best for our patients.

Successive governments have introduced guidelines, legislation and mandates to ensure that NHS staff behave in particular ways: treat patients more or less; work in new ways; cut out ways of working that we may fundamentally

5 Swinburn K. Journeys with aphasia: personal reflections. In: Anderson C, Van der Gagg A, editors. *Speech and Language Therapy: issues in professional practice*. Whurr Publishers Ltd; 2005. Ch. 7, p. 127.

6 Norwood G. *Maslow's Hierarchy of Needs. The truth vectors (Part I)*. [1999], retrieved June 2012. Available at: www.deepermind.com/20maslow.htm (accessed April 2013).

believe in, to our very core. We may be asked to practise remotely, to deliver treatment indirectly; to delegate parts of our work to less qualified people. We are more frequently, particularly in the present climate, asked to add to our workload, for example, weave public health messages into our work with patients.

In this chapter I will begin by exploring some of the ways we can, as healthcare workers, begin to develop our clinical thinking, to sharpen up our ideas on the way some of the government messages can be challenged, for the best benefit of our patients. In the second part of the chapter, I will give some examples of how to put these new ways of working into practice with patients/clients.

Challenging the agenda

To grow professionally, we must never take 'orders' at face value: we are expected to think, to ask questions, to raise doubts, to challenge. We must dare to confront. We must be assertive in our responses. For instance, over the last decade many front line workers have – as part of their normal working day – been asked to advise their patients about their weight, smoking and drinking habits. Initially, the message was opportunistic, so if the patient happened to consult on that issue we could issue advice. Then, with the advent of GP targets, health workers were required to record details of body mass index, smoking and drinking habits. In 2011, the media picked up on one of the key planks of this message: it was suggested that, regardless of the reason for consultation, health workers, as partners in supporting change, should advice on weight management/smoking cessation/alcohol misuse if the patient was noted to have any of those presenting problems. Here we look at the weight management strategy set out in the White Paper, *Healthy Lives, Healthy People: our strategy for public health in England*, in more detail.[7]

The problem with this is simply that telling the patient they need to lose weight/stop smoking/stop drinking does not work. We have seen that for change to occur, we need ownership, and for change to be managed, we need to work closely on behavioural change and motivational factors. Of course, the full government message, embedded in the White Paper, is not simplistic; it does look at a variety of factors that need to change, and looks at the best ways to implement these. However, for the busy healthcare worker, seeing patients about issues other than weight, for example, time and personal competence are big issues for the worker. Many healthcare workers are not trained to deliver such powerful, personal messages. Many will not even have considered their own issues around body image, or value judgements about size. Because of this,

---

7 Department of Health. *Healthy Lives, Healthy People: our strategy for public health in England*. Cm. 7985. Department of Health; 2010.

the majority will struggle to get the message over in such a way that supports and empowers the patient to make the changes needed themselves.

Here we consider the kind of approaches that we need, the type of treatment package that we need to apply where we want the patient/client to change their behaviour in some way. This can include the changes needed to become more assertive, to eat or drink less, to take medication regularly or to do the exercises prescribed. We need to think more broadly about the ways we manage our patients, incorporating a more managed care approach to treatment. To help us unpick this, let us stay with, and consider how, we could support someone in changing their eating habits.

Changing eating habits

The government is rightly concerned about the levels of obesity in the UK. The latest Health Survey for England data[8] shows that nearly one in four adults and over one in 10 children aged between two and 10 are obese. We know that obesity can have a severe impact on people's health, increasing the risk of type 2 diabetes, some cancers, and heart and liver disease. There is also a significant burden on the NHS – direct costs caused by obesity are estimated to be £4.2 billion per year and forecast to more than double by 2050 if we carry on as we are. Reducing obesity is a priority for the government. It wants people to think that they can change their lifestyle and make a difference to their health. The message in the White Paper is:

> 'The Government will provide clear, consistent messages on why people should change their lifestyle, how to do so, and put in place ways to make this easier … by encouraging them to eat well, move more and live longer.'

In highlighting this section of the White Paper, I want to begin applying some of the strategies we have learnt about so far. The message above is a medical model message at its worst. It is authoritarian and patronising. It delivers a professional opinion which demeans patients and makes them unequal in the relationship. It is neither empowering, nor self-educating. There are many overweight people who already know they are overweight (and, if women, exactly how overweight). They do not need their GP to tell them this, nor *how* to diet and exercise. Many overweight people already know that crisps and cake are 'bad' and fruit and veg are 'good'. The *should* is redundant.

If we work with a social model, we understand that a client's experience is placed within a broader societal context. Our role then is work with the

---

8 Zaninotto P, Wardle H, Stamatakis E, *et al. Forecasting Obesity to 2010*. Joint Health Surveys Unit, National Centre for Social Research, Department of Epidemiology and Public Health, Royal Free and University College Medical School; 2010.

individual to understand the impact of the problem – if it is a problem for the patient – and address any context-driven issues of importance to their life. Within this, we as the clinicians, can be used as a resource, the facilitators who inform but do not lead the process of change. The change belongs to the service user, not us.

Thus, we need to find out how much the overweight person understands and feels about the 'shoulds' and 'oughts'. How do they feel about their size? Authoritarian messages carry judgement, and that judgement may evoke feelings of being bad, different, greedy, out of control, lazy or humiliation. In this space the person may not feel comfortable about sharing their knowledge of the several 'diets' they have been on, all of which curtailed certain foods or food groups and can be seen as a way of handling eating and bodily difficulties by another name.[9] Many overweight people absolutely know what they should do, but they are not doing it. And why not is what needs to be considered and acknowledged. We have an odd cultural relationship with food here in the West. For example, the fact we fetishise and loathe it simultaneously; the paradox of surrounding ourselves with images of delicious food while simultaneously lauding the desirability of extreme thinness in people. This type of thinking needs to be reflected in government recommendations.

We have identified that most of our decision making has in the past been clinically driven, based on the condition, not the presenting circumstances. To help us move on from this, we know we need to work collaboratively with the client/patient to unpick the presenting problem. To support this way of working, we can use models of change such as Motivational Interviewing and the Transtheoretical model (spiral of change). We could change our questioning to support the patient in their thinking.

➤ 'How do you think I can help?'
➤ 'What can I offer you that is new?'
➤ 'Has something changed?'
➤ 'If so, how can I help now?'

There is acknowledgement in the White Paper of wider thinking and long-term working and planning.
➤ Partnership working with local government, charities and business to reduce obesity and to strengthen both national and local leadership.
➤ Promoting Change4Life: England's national social marketing campaign to promote healthy weight. But it aims to prevent people from becoming overweight by using the above encouraging message.
➤ A partnership between the Department of Health and the Association of

---

9 Orbach S. *Bodies*. Profile Books; 2009. p. 97.

Convenience Stores to increase the availability of fresh fruit and vegetables in areas that might otherwise have limited access to them.

➤ A National Child Measurement Programme uses the information gained to help the NHS and local authorities plan and provide better health services for children.

➤ A recognition that the advertising and marketing of food to children can influence food habits. The government will continue to work with Ofcom and the Advertising Standards Authority to ensure healthier foods are promoted in the media.

➤ A Childhood Obesity National Support Team, established in 2007 to assist local areas in improving the quality and impact of healthy weight delivery systems and interventions. It supports local areas in addressing unhealthy behaviours that lead to excess weight gain during pregnancy, in children and young people, and in their families. It has helped to steer local areas towards actions that improve the quality and interventions and to create environments that support individuals and families to lead healthier lives.

This is looking better, but it is not enough. The government has clearly demonstrated its thinking around some of the environmental and cultural changes needed to support people with their weight loss targets. But what is sadly missing from the White Paper is some of the psychological references, some recognition of the psychological management required, which is unusual given the very detailed and evidenced-based work the government has undertaken on alcohol and substance abuse programmes.

Does encouragement work?

Telling or encouraging someone that they need to lose weight, for example, does not take into account the cultural and individual complexity of our relationship with food, weight, body image. Consider how this message accounts for the following examples.

➤ Any individual and unique motivating factors that would support required change, such as goals, moral rules, laws, social expectations, personal commitments and other forces.

➤ Known facts about motivation. Psychologists say that two traits are likely to make us more successful at achieving set targets: high intelligence and self-control (the ability to change thoughts, emotions, actions and level of performance on duties and tasks).[10]

➤ Willpower. Research shows repeatedly that after people exert self-control, they tend to perform relatively poorly on a subsequent, seemingly irrelevant test of self-control. It is as if we 'use up' a bit of our willpower as

---

10 Baumeister R. Where has your willpower gone? *New Scientist*. 2012 Jan 28. pp. 30–31.

we go, leaving us less likely to be able to resist temptation as the day wears on: it is the cumulative exertion that saps the willpower. If you do not have many temptations to resist, your willpower can stay relatively strong. Self-control weakens but can be replenished after a rest.[11] We need to examine how this enables the dieter to manage their diet throughout the day, and it may be one of the main factors in diet recidivism rates.

➤ Willpower is 'domain general': controlling thoughts, emotions and feelings, restraining impulses, performing tasks and duties will draw on one pool of willpower, not multiple pools with different quantities for, say, diet or exercise. Other interesting work shows, paradoxically, that in order to resist temping foods, we need willpower, but to have willpower we must eat. The essence of dieting (restricting food intake) robs us of the psychological strength needed to succeed.[12] We need to examine how this enables the dieter to manage their diet/exercise regime.

➤ Any individual and unique genetic/metabolic/health issues that make weight gain more or less likely, and affect size, depend on a transformation of personal biology.

➤ The 24-hour availability of easily obtainable, cheap, unhealthy 'food' in express stores, garages, supermarkets and fridges throughout the country, which make it very hard to maintain lifelong resistance: imagine if street drugs, equally addictive and tempting to some, were so obtainable.

➤ The cultural pervasion of technology, which has changed many of us into sedentary, computer-based people at work.

➤ Too little time means we choose the car not the bus, and the bus not walking, to get from A to B.

➤ The cultural norms that mean the provision of food equals nurture and hospitality (plus an addictive boost of oxytocin to the provider).

➤ The built in sense of 'otherness' fostered by cultural norms of 'thinness' 'beauty', 'fitness' and the media exposure/pressure to conform to this. Do not assume these are shared values: ask.

➤ The conflicting media messages – the relentless advertising of industrialised, processed, packaged food – alongside adverts for diet products.

➤ How is the 'encouraging' health worker going to help their client manage any feelings of deprivation? Temptation?

➤ Companies that produce diet products rely on a 95% recidivism rate.[13] Difficult feelings of anger, anxiety, self-hatred and disgust emerge when the desired weight loss does not happen as quickly as desired, or at all,

---

11 Ibid.
12 Ibid.
13 Orbach, note 9 above, p. 97.

or is reversed when the 'diet' is complete. To see the pounds coming off can give a feeling of pride and success, a real achievement. There is a temporary feeling better as the incentive/resource seeking feeling blocks out the unpleasant feelings from the threat/self-protection system. There is a good feeling of control, which evaporates with weight gain, or is reinforced with continued weight loss, as demonstrated by anorexic behaviours.[14]

➤ The need to manage the changing relationship with the body as it changes size, and other people behave differently towards the thinner person, not always positively – sometimes angrily, enviously. Our relationship with food and body image is so complex and pervasive that many people in close relationship with the 'dieter' consciously or unconsciously sabotage their efforts to lose weight.

➤ We all have enormous and often unconscious value judgements about size. Many feel free to make direct and personal comments on someone's size in ways that would be considered unacceptable in other arenas ('Oh, your skin is so black!', 'How come you use a wheelchair?). This can lead the recipient of the comments to feel exposed, vulnerable and self-conscious. We need to take responsibility for invoking these feelings as we put our client's very selves under scrutiny, and judge so harshly.

➤ What does 'food' mean to the client/patient? Is it used as a reward? To nurture? To block feelings? If so, there is a need to help break the link between food as a source of comfort, reward and solace, if the production of feel-good endorphins/opiates such as oxytocin may no longer be produced.

➤ How to help support the mother who needs to nurture and feed her child and family every mealtime (but not herself)? What can she feed herself to feel 'held' in this time?

➤ What about the client's family history of food; the messages around food given by their mother especially – what is her relationship to food? What messages were they given about food as a child? Was it plentiful, available, denied, did they feel deprived, loved, nurtured through food?

➤ If an unhappy relationship to food and body size exists, confusions and ambivalence are created around size and food. It may be that a fatter body is being used, consciously or unconsciously, as a challenging statement to a parent, society or consumerism.

➤ For those who are considered either too fat or too thin (and this is a value judgement), it is common not to know when one is hungry or sated. The sense of having a stable body whose size and appetites one knows can

14 Gilbert P. *The Compassionate Mind*. Kindle ed. Constable; 2010. p. 176.

be elusive. Where this ambivalence and confusion exist, there can be no peace.[15]

All this complexity needs to be acknowledged and managed. There can be an addiction to food, but, unlike alcohol or drugs, it is not possible to stop eating. There can be no sudden stopping, no ability not to go to pubs or clubs or the places where there is no food, as food is everywhere, and we all have to eat it three times a day. How to help the patient manage this? It is clear that more than a reprimand and 'encouragement' are needed. When these questions are considered, the government message looks not only foolish but impossible. People do not change because they are told to do so. People must not only want to change, but must also give themselves the reasons to make the change bearable, possible. They have to have more reasons to change than not, and they need help, support and guidance to effect the changes.

Of course, we need to guide and support our clients/patients in focussing about what they want to achieve over the long and short term, and be specific about the losses and gains. We need to support them in the work: to look at the outcome they want to achieve and also be clear about what they want to do towards achieving their goal on a daily basis. But it is their work, not ours. We help facilitate the change; it does not belong to us.

MANAGING THE CHANGE

We have established that for change to occur it has to be owned, and the underlying complexities unpicked and understood. As Malcomess has established,[16] we cannot apply the same care pathways mechanically to all clients within the same diagnostic group, as care is driven by impact and risk to the individual, not to the diagnostic group. Here we look through some of the ideas we explored in Chapter 4, Putting your ideas into practice, but this time the focus is on the patient/client, not ourselves. These ideas can be used to support patients through any behavioural change, from becoming more assertive, changing eating habits, stopping smoking or drinking, to trying out a new exercise regime. Many practitioners (therapists, mental health team practitioners, drug and alcohol teams) need to teach assertiveness skills directly: these ideas can be a useful adjunct.

---

15 Orbach, note 9 above, p. 100.
16 Malcomess K. The Care Aims model. In: Anderson C, van der Gaag A, editors. *Speech and Language Therapy: issues in professional practice*. Whurr Publishers Ltd; 2005.

Goal setting

1   Lifetime goals

Thinking about what they want to achieve over the long and short term helps people to break their thinking down a little more to be specific about the losses and gains that achieving this goal will bring. Look carefully at the outcome they want to achieve, and also be clear about what they want to do towards achieving their goal on a daily basis. Here is the model we looked at in Chapter 2, taken from *Neurolinguistic Programming for Dummies,*[17] adapted for use with those we help.

Where are you now?

Consider individually with the client/patient what it is they actually want to change and why. If they do not want to change, abandon the work (revisit the Spiral of change transtheoretical health model in the last chapter: *see* pages 187–8). Use whatever clinical indicators are needed: smoking, drinking, managing medication or pain. However, not that many of the life areas overlap, so choose those that are most relevant. For example, if you want to support your client/patient with weight loss, look at all the areas identified in the examples below, as weight loss would have a big impact on all. In the second column, I suggest some of these questions that may be useful for these 'addiction' type behaviours. Ask the patient/client how happy they are with these areas of their life, using a score of 1 to 10.

EXAMPLE 1

Influencing factors

Health and fitness/exercise
1...2...3...4...5...6...7...8...9...10
Friendships /family and support networks
1...2...3...4...5...6...7...8...9...10
Rest and relaxation
1...2...3...4...5...6...7...8...9...10
Health/eating/weight
1...2...3...4...5...6...7...8...9...10

---

17 Ready R, Burton K. *Neurolinguistic Programming for Dummies.* John Wiley & Sons; 2004. Ch. 3, pp. 36–45, Taking charge of your life.

Stress management

1...2...3...4...5...6...7...8...9...10

If I were thinner/fatter/pain free/could walk to the shops/drive I would

....

EXAMPLE 2

Factors influencing diet

Use these questions as a springboard to develop more understanding about your client's relationship with food and their body. Many women in particular have an ingrained fear of appetite and an unreliable body sense, despite striving for thin-ness and being afraid of managing it.[18]

Who are you doing this for?
Score 10 if you want these changes for yourself; score 1 if it is for someone else (a partner, a friend, the doctor)
1...2...3...4...5...6...7...8...9...10

How important is your body image to you?
1...2...3...4...5...6...7...8...9...10

Do you eat with appetite, and finish when sated?
Use this scale to explore how 'in touch' the client is with their body. A low score may indicate if food represents something other than fuel/nutrition.
1...2...3...4...5...6...7...8...9...10

What sorts of foods do you tend to prefer?
Use 1 = healthy/unprocessed and 10= snacks, processed, industrialised foods
1...2...3...4...5...6...7...8...9...10

Any individual medical or family history that makes weight gain more or less likely?
1= none, 10 = high influence
1...2...3...4...5...6...7...8...9...10

Are you easily influenced by advertising or food availability?
1...2...3...4...5...6...7...8...9...10

Is it easy to incorporate increased exercise into your current lifestyle?
1...2...3...4...5...6...7...8...9...10

Do you have to provide food for family/friends on a regular basis?
1...2...3...4...5...6...7...8...9...10

18 Orbach, note 9 above, p. 100.

Do you feel pressured by cultural norms of 'thinness', 'beauty', 'fitness'?
1…2…3…4…5…6…7…8…9…10

Do you think your family history has a bearing here?
What messages did you receive from your family about body image?
1…2…3…4…5…6…7…8…9…10

Do you feel defensive and judged when food is a topic of conversation?
1…2…3…4…5…6…7…8…9…10

How many diets have you been on in the past?
1…2…3…4…5…6…7…8…9…10

Have they worked? For how long? What stopped them working?
1…2…3…4…5…6…7…8…9…10

Do you have any difficult feelings if you weigh yourself and have not lost weight?
1…2…3…4…5…6…7…8…9…10

How often do you weigh yourself?
1= never, 10 = twice daily
1…2…3…4…5…6…7…8…9…10

How often do you self-check?
1…2…3…4…5…6…7…8…9…10

Who can you identify as the best support for your plan?
Note each friend/family member and be honest about the level of support they can give you, with 1= none and 10= 100% unconditional practical and emotional help
1…2…3…4…5…6…7…8…9…10

Do you 'use' food for emotional sustenance, or simply eat to live?
For 'eat to live' =1, for use of food as emotional sustenance = 10.
1…2…3…4…5…6…7…8…9…10

Already you have begun to unpick some of the issues that need addressing. You have broadened your, and your patient's, perspective on the presenting issues, and now you need to begin to set goals.

Setting the goals

1 Lifetime goals

Having noted where they are now, note what they want to achieve over a lifetime. What number do you think is attainable? What about 10 years? Five years?

2   Short-term goals

Now consider the short-term goals – more tangible, six months to one year, perhaps.

➤ Make them SMART (see below).

➤ Make sure it is initiated, maintained and within the client's own control

➤ They must be stated positively 'I will', 'I can …'

➤ Check whether the goals are within their control to effect.

➤ Describe the content: 'Who/why/what/where/when can this be achieved?', 'What will I want to do with it?'

➤ Does the goal identify any required resources? People? Money? Time?

➤ Does it identify the first step they need to take?

➤ Ask how they will let you know the outcome? 'How will I see it, smell it, hear or feel it?'

➤ Will there be any secondary gains? 'How will this benefit the environment, my family, friends?', 'Will I save money,? 'Who else will be happy?'

➤ Ask them to make a list of the losses and gains if they achieve their goal (*see* motivational interviewing, below).

➤ What would happen if they achieved their goal, and if they do not? Make that list.

Your client will need extrinsic rewards: give them targets to achieve and record, and revisit it regularly. Discuss ways to keep them focussed on the benefits of success. Ask them what they will use to reward themselves.

3   SMART goals

Refer back to the setting of goals in Chapter 4. Patients, like us, need something to work towards, to help them feel they are moving along a specific path. Once we have established some of the motivating factors, establishing goals invites us to look at the big picture, to break it down into smaller pieces and get started towards accomplishing our important hopes and dreams. Set the scene for the patient. Explain that many people are not quite sure how to set goals, and that one of the most common problems is that their goals tend to be too big. It is much easier to achieve smaller goals that fit with a larger objective than to try to accomplish everything all at once. So that the goal setting becomes more manageable, use the SMART technique to help you define these goals: All targets, aims, objectives and the reinforcers/rewards you use must be SMART.

S   Be *Specific* – the goals must be clear and concrete: 'I will drink a glass of water every meal time.'

M   Make sure the goals are *Measurable* and *Motivating*: identify markers that will indicate when the goals have been reached. If you are working through a programme with a patient, this may be through standardised assessments or standardised objectives.

A   *Achievable* – ensure that the goals are realistic. Check and double check with the patient/client whether their goal is achievable or not.

R   *Relevant/Realistic* – choose goals that are applicable to the patient's personal development. Make sure that these goals are something they are truly invested in, because you will be focusing a great deal of time and energy on them.

T   *Time-related* – set a timeline that will guide their progress, make it *Timely*: set a relevant timeline that is powerful and motivating.

Specifying a goal for two years down the road is not as powerful a motivator as one that you set for the next six months.

SMART goals do not necessarily have to be about the patient's achievements; they may also be about the environment to allow the patient to access/improve/ function.

For any behavioural change to be effective, the work has to be very focused. Whoever is teaching the skills has to communicate the stages of the work very clearly and ensure that the parents/carers/patients understand the importance of setting clear boundaries for the treatment to be effective. When teaching a new skill, or making any lifestyle change, – going on a diet, reducing drinking, following an exercise programme, doing pelvic floor exercises etc. – the when, how, who, where, what considerations outlined previously need to be taken into account.

Collect together ideas of age-appropriate privileges/treats/rewards to help patients learn to control their own behaviour in order to gain a reward (e.g. for a child, collect tokens), and be clear about rules, rewards and consequences. Write them up and display them. If you are working on habit change, support patients with a diary or success chart to help keep them motivated:

Try one new idea every day

Date	Activity	Marks out of 10	Comments

WORKING WITH RESISTANCE

There may be many reasons for people finding it hard to change, some of which we have identified above. Before we discuss resistance as a factor, it may be worth exploring some of the other factors that contribute to a high level of risk in clients, outlined by Malcomess:[19]

➤ client/carer's awareness/understanding of the condition and its risks
➤ client/carer's capacity to manage risk (historically and in the present)
➤ client/carer's willingness to take responsibility for risk
➤ client's insight
➤ environmental factors, for example, social context, skills and capacity of carers, cultural considerations, etc.
➤ time of onset
➤ client's life circumstances, for example, age, employment status, responsibility for dependants, level of social interaction needed, education potential, etc.
➤ direct impact of the condition, for example, on physical health, feelings, functional ability
➤ indirect impact of the condition, for example, on the effectiveness of other treatment
➤ concern of others.

The motivational interviewing approach is very useful if people are non-compliant or very anxious, or to highlight a discrepancy between their motivation that of and their partner/helper/carer. If the consultation is proving to be challenging, and the patient is demanding outside help but not taking personal responsibility for their part in making necessary changes, these techniques may be helpful. This can also be useful to identify both the skill level of the patient and whether they actually want to work on their needs.

We know that for change to occur, there needs to be more positives than negatives about making the change. If there are more negatives, it is unlikely that the goal will be achieved, and this needs to be discussed. However, if the patient is using lots of 'change talk', for example, 'I *am going to* do X', this is good sign that change will occur. Give examples of positives and negatives as a guide. Here is a brief guide to the questioning that needs to happen to ensure that you have gained their motivation.

A typical day
What does a typical day look like? At home, school, family time, etc.

---

19 Malcomess, note 16 above.

Information exchange

Is there anything about your illness/functional skills, etc. that you are unhappy about?

How important is it to work on this?

On a scale of 1 to 10, what number would you give yourself right now?

0 Not at all important.. 10 very important

Can you explain why you have given yourself this number?
Why did you not give yourself a lower number?
What could you do to move yourself up the scale?

If you did decide to work on this, how confident are you that you would succeed?

On a scale of 1 to 10, what number would you give yourself right now?

0 Not at all confident...10 very confident

Can you explain why you have given yourself this number?
Why did you not give yourself a lower number?
What could you do to move yourself up the scale?

What might be the *not* so good things about developing these skills/giving up X/walking well, etc.?

What might be the *good* things about developing these skills/giving up X/walking well, etc.?

The experimental record sheet

Another way to support patients with change is for them actually to try out some of the new behaviours – test run them – and record what has happened. This would be an ideal treatment for the particularly nervous patient, or those with low self-esteem, those who avoid, those who are passive or those who are lacking in confidence.

We looked at the following strategies in Chapter 4, and here they have been re-worked. The principles are taken from cognitive behaviour therapy. Individual and group treatment programmes can be used to help patients change their behaviour/faulty thinking by testing their predictions of failure/ disaster and discovering what actually happens. If you feel comfortable with the model, skip this section.

Challenging negative beliefs

Here you encourage your patient or client to note whether they have a negative belief ('I will never be able to do X'). Encourage them to challenge this belief through experimenting with it.

How much you believe this. 10%? 50%? 85%?

Now challenge or dispute this belief. Take it apart. How accurate is it? Get to the facts.

Challenging the belief

Examine the evidence for and against.

Evidence for

➤ What makes you think you could never do this?
➤ How does not doing this help you cope or solve the problem?
➤ Where is the evidence for this belief?
➤ Is it good, solid and reliable evidence?
➤ Is there any other way you could view this evidence for yourself?

Evidence against

➤ Have there been times when you have acted in these circumstances?
➤ What are the disadvantages of not acting?
➤ Have there been situations when you have acted, and it all turned out ok?
➤ What actually happened? What are the facts?

Ask your patients to keep a record of their experiments, so in discussion with you they can test their own hypothesis and see if their predictions were true. Give information about brain chemistry that explains why we tend to believe more in our negative than our positive predictions about the world, and explain why it is important to appraise a situation accurately.

Here is another way you could encourage your client to record their practice.

1 Prediction

Outline the thought or belief you are testing and rate the patient's strength of conviction between 0 and 100%.

2 Experiment

Experiment with the patient, and plan what exactly it is they will do. Be very specific and include *what* they will do, *who* they will do it with, and *where*, *when* and *how*. Consider any obstacles, and how they will be overcome. Plan what to do if the prediction comes true, for example, how will they respond assertively if someone sneers at them, or argues with them? Think how you will measure the results.

3   Record the results

Make a note of what actually happened, using clear, observable outcomes. Include the thoughts, feelings, any physical sensations and what the other people did. As the patient describes what they are feeling, they increase frontal lobe regulation of the limbic system, enabling them to feel calmer and in control.

4   Conclusion

Use this column to record their conclusion and write any comments. Evaluate the results. What have they learned about their predictions? Were they accurate? Has their theory changed in light of the results? Re-rate their original strength of conviction in percentage terms.

5   The future

Plan ways the for the patient to consolidate what they have discovered. For example, should they repeat it, try another one? Do it differently? Try to stretch them to try a new way.

Already you can see this is a very different way of working with people to achieve change. The medical model dictates that we prescribe and tell; here we are empowering, giving patients the power to make choices and changes in their life. We are allowing them the space and giving them the tools to help facilitate the changes; we are helping to guide, steer and support change, not to direct it. It is a very different way of working, and one that many of us will not feel comfortable with initially, but it is the only way to facilitate long-term change in people's behaviour.

THE SHORT-CUT METHOD

This new way of working does take time, and cannot be embarked on unless there is the time and space to do so. However, it is possible to short-cut many of the techniques, and by some judicious questioning help the patient/client to begin to adjust to the idea of taking responsibility for, and planning their own, changes. Here are some suggestions. Take what would work for you in the time frame available to you and try some of them out.

How important is it to work on this?
On a scale of 1 to 10, what number would you give yourself right now?

0 Not at all important... 10 very important

Can you explain why you have given yourself this number?
Why did you not give yourself a lower number?
What could you do to move yourself up the scale?

Setting goals

What is the *lifetime goal*? The *short-term goal*? Their *reward system*?
Are the goals *SMART*?
Discuss *when*, *where* and *who* to work with?

Challenging negative beliefs

What is the evidence for, and the evidence against, this belief?
Plan what exactly it is they will do. Be very specific and include *what* they will do, *who* they will do it with, *where*, *when* and *how*. What have they learned about their predictions? Were they accurate?

On a scale of 1 to 10

Who are you doing this for?
How important is it to do it?
How easy will it be to incorporate it into your current lifestyle?
How many times have you tried this in the past? What happened?
What stopped it working and how is it different now?
Who can you identify as the best support for your plan?
Where and *when* will you do X?

KEY POINTS

➤ We need to work reflectively, assertively, to challenge the status quo and ourselves: to move out of our usual comfort zone, exploring unchartered waters that may provoke uncomfortable feelings. Our personal development and professional accountability demand that we listen, but always question, and apply any recommendations with due intelligence, confidence, assertiveness and consideration for what is best for our patients.

➤ We need to support our clients with changing – their sense of self, their skills – and to know how to motivate and support them with making these changes.

➤ We need to understand our clients' expectations and their perspective on both their condition and the service we offer, and only then can we move forward into a care partnership of shared decision making.

➤ In conversation, the transaction is the more obvious, overt, verbal element; the interaction the hidden, covert element. Throughout the process of supporting our patients to see things differently, to learn and change, we need to hold awareness of these overt and covert methods of communicating.

➤ Getting people to open up and confide in us is a real skill. If the patient or client has a story they need to tell, and you need to hear, they need to be able to trust that you will 'hold' the information safely and support them without judgement. We do this through allowing time to build up trust, telling the truth, reflecting, allowing feelings so that a coherent narrative can be built. We hold our own feelings in check.

➤ We all have the right to remain silent: when it is unsafe to disclose we may feel unhappy, vulnerable and exposed. It may be more important quietly to accept the unsaid.

➤ How much do our responses convey an understanding of the client's experience? How well do our responses reflect the essence of what our client is communicating? How well are we responsively attuned? Are we 'directing' the client, rather than following their lead?

➤ We need to develop the core skills of being non-judgmental, and to demonstrate warm positive regard. We need to be able to 'hold' the client in their distress. We need to collaborate on how much the therapist appropriately and skilfully works to facilitate new awareness, growth and self-determination and empowerment in the client.

➤ Part of the therapeutic role is to encourage people to see themselves in relation to their problem, instead of simply having the problem. This leads naturally to a more positive approach, to externalising rather than internalising and personalising the problem.

➤ People may have different information and motivation needs at different stages. They may seek information to help them cope, in order to meet their basic needs. They may seek information to help them feel safe and secure. They may seek to be enlightened or empowered.

➤ People have to 'own' the changes, they have to be in charge of them.

➤ Part of being assertive, too, is to be courageous in challenging agendas that are set for us by others. Our work in healthcare is impacted by government and management agendas, and we may not always agree. We grow through listening, questioning and applying any recommendations with due intelligence, confidence, assertiveness and consideration for what is best for our patients. To grow professionally, we must never take 'orders' at face value: we are expected to think, to ask questions, to raise doubts, to challenge. We must dare to confront.

➤ The medical model at its worst is authoritarian and patronising. It delivers a professional opinion which demeans patients and makes them unequal in the relationship. It is neither empowering nor self-educating. We need to move towards being used as a resource – the facilitators who inform but do not lead the process of change. The change belongs to the service user, not us.

➤ Any individual, and unique, motivating factors that would support required change. This may include goals, moral rules, laws, social expectations, personal commitments and other forces.

➤ Thinking about what they want to achieve over the long and short term helps patients to break their thinking down a little more, to be specific about the losses and gains that achieving this goal will bring. Look carefully at the outcome they want to achieve, and also be clear about what they want to do toward achieving their goal on a daily basis.

➤ SMART goals do not necessarily have to be about the patient's achievements; they may also be about the environment to allow the patient to access/improve/function.

➤ For any behavioural change to be effective, the work has to be very focussed. Whoever is teaching the skills has to communicate the stages of the work very clearly and ensure that the parents/carers/patients understand the importance of setting clear boundaries for the treatment to be effective.

➤ Some of the actors that contribute to a high level of risk in clients are the client's insight, environmental/social factors, awareness/understanding of the condition, their capacity to manage risk and willingness to take responsibility for risk, the direct and indirect impact of the condition, and the support of others.

➤ The motivational interviewing approach is very useful if patients are non-compliant, challenging or very anxious, or to highlight a discrepancy between the motivation of the patient and their partner/helper/carer.

Challenging negative beliefs. What is the evidence for, and the evidence against, this belief? Plan what exactly it is they will do. Be very specific. What have they learned about their predictions? Were they accurate?

FURTHER READING

Nathan P, Smith L, Rees C, *et al. Mood Management Course: a cognitive behavioural group treatment programme for anxiety and depression.* 2nd ed. Centre for Clinical Interventions; 2004. Available at: www.cci.health.wa.gov.au/ (accessed April 2013).

CHAPTER 13

Breaking unwelcome news

Among the most difficult conversations that healthcare professionals have with their patients are discussions around the end of treatment. Although practitioners/clinicians may perceive a discharge to be positive, for many reasons or our clients and patients may not, so we need to be aware of the need to be careful, constructive and compassionate in our communications at this time. End of care conversations can range from a 'good' discharge, where the treatment ends normally and the patient's needs are fully met, to unwanted discussions around end of life care, terminal illnesses and degenerative conditions. Our NHS values spell out our need to treat people with respect and dignity, to commit to quality of care, to improve lives with compassion and to work inclusively, without excluding anyone or any group. There are times when the need to be intuitive, empathic and assertive – using clear, honest and open communications – is courageous and crucial.

Any one of us may need to say:
➤ the recommended treatments for this condition are no longer working
➤ the side effects may on balance, spoil your quality of life
➤ there is no more – or effective – treatment for your condition.

In this chapter we are examining the best ways to communicate 'bad', or unwanted, news.

The news will of itself be in a range: from the unwanted news to the client of a counsellor that her six allotted treatments are up, to delivering the news that there is no cure for a life-threatening or life-limiting condition. There are some groups of patients for whom any news is going to be perceived as additionally threatening, because of their own life story, medical history or mental health issues. Clinical experience shows that, in particular, parents of children can be very demanding, and are often unhappy if what they value as treatment options are withdrawn or withheld. Their role is to advocate for their child, and they are going to want the very best for that child. We are also aware of those with an acute dread of illness, whose own anxiety will pull them into an acute fear response with the mildest of news.

As humans, we struggle to face the unknown, we like to feel we are in control of our destinies, and have yet to confront fully the processes of managing uncertainty, illness, difficulty, disability, through to having more control in the process of our deaths. Although we find this difficult, possibly because of our fears surrounding the subject, the way we deal with disability and death in our society is often far from compassionate. Medicine can prolong both, which is not the same as prolonging life. The challenge here, as workers close to illness and the process of dying, is to recognise the importance of kindness and affection and compassion, and place these qualities at the centre of our dealings with patients as they face their personal tragedies.

It has been suggested that the NHS can be considered as a receptacle for the nation's fears of death, a system to shield us from the anxieties arising from an awareness of illness and mortality.[1] Similarly, Hoggett has argued that public institutions, in addition to their explicit goals, are often required to contain what is disowned by the rest of society: in this way, they become an arena for the contestability of public concerns and purposes via the projection of unconscious desires and conflicts in society.

This may help to explain the outrage in developed countries when advanced medical technologies cannot be made available to all; or the unfounded hopes in experimental treatments; or the tendency to feel duped when interventions fail. In all these situations, both individuals and society at large are quick to blame, as if good enough medical care should prevent illness and death. Patients and doctors collude in this to prevent the former from facing their fear of death and the latter from facing their fallibility. We too, as clinicians, are recruited into the fantasy of protecting us from our own mortality.

In this chapter too we begin to unpick some of our own ethical and moral values. Ethical values do have a social context and are exemplified by honesty, integrity and loyalty. Competence values include creativity, flexibility and patience,[2] all of which help the individual to achieve their best, in and out of work. Here we look at some of the ways healthcare professionals, particularly but not exclusively doctors, can be helped to become more sensitive to the patient perspective, and to the patient's desire to be respected, and cared for. Poor communication between patients and their doctors can contribute to poor adherence to the care management. Successful user involvement means, among other things:

---

1 Obholzer A. Managing social anxieties in public sector organizations. In: Reynolds J, Henderson J, Seden J, *et al.*, editors. *The Managing Care Reader*. Routledge; 2003. pp. 281–8. Hoggett P. Pity, compassion, solidarity. In: Clarke S, Hoggett P, Thompson S, editors. *Emotions, Politics and Society*. Palgrave Macmillan; 2006. pp. 145–61. Rizq R. IAPT, anxiety and envy: a psychoanalytic view of NHS primary care mental health services today. *British Journal of Psychotherapy*. 2011; **27**(1): 37–55.

2 Anderson C, van der Gaag A, editors. *Speech and Language Therapy: issues in professional practice*. Whurr Publishers Ltd; 2005.

➤ the provision of clear information
➤ encouraging the patient to ask questions
➤ willingness to share decisions and agreement between patient and professional about the problems and the plan.[3]

It is never easy to communicate bad news, however much we practise and prepare for it. Before anything is said, we need to be made aware of some of the possible and principal *causes* of conflict in this scenario:
➤ miscommunications, misunderstandings, personality clashes
➤ poor understanding on the part of the clinician about the exact personal history and personality of the patient
➤ a potential culture clash – acute, secondary sector clinicians are almost always scientists, with a very linear, pragmatic way of thinking; the soft art of communicating with their patient may be counter-intuitive for them
➤ different understandings between the patient and clinician about the clinical detail, the rationale, goals and methods used
➤ problems relating to misunderstandings about areas of responsibility ('But I thought you were the ones who had the authority to prescribe X!')
➤ competition for limited resources
➤ non-compliance with, or avoidance of, rules or policies
➤ different understandings of material communicated between the communicator and the receiver, when the receiver is in a state of shock
➤ different ways of working, and different paperwork used, throughout the NHS.

To make it easier for the NHS to deliver unwanted news, patient expectations and the perceived culture of the NHS needs to change. While people expect treatment always to end in cure, and medicine to be delivered paternalistically, without patient engagement or effort, we in the NHS will always be raised on a dais of our own making. While the public perceive that the NHS will give whatever is needed for as long as is needed, expectations run high, so any news of discharge or inability/unwillingness to help is seen on a continuum from meanness to an admission of failure; both very uncomfortable places to work from.

THE FIRST STEP: WHAT TO COMMUNICATE

First and foremost, patients quite rightly need good, unbiased, well-delivered information about their choices, and to be prepared – forewarned – about the limits of any treatment so that expectations are not raised unnecessarily.

---

3 Stewart M. Studies of health outcomes and patient centered communication. In: Stewart M, Brown J, Weston W, *et al.*, editors. *Patient Centered Medicine*. Sage; 1995.

In this way, many of the above situations (miscommunications, different understandings about goals/methods, misunderstandings about areas of responsibility) are avoided. One way (of many) to solve this is to give as much information about the condition/profession/treatment as possible, preferably verbally, definitely backed up in writing, given that most people find it hard to remember detail when they are stressed or distracted. The example below is one delivered to parents of children undergoing therapy in the community, a primary care setting. It could be used as a basis for discussion, shared understanding of goals, or to form a contract of care. Incorporated in the model are some concepts about motivation and change management, taken from taken from the Transtheoretical model of change.[4]

How we work

These approaches are used to help you and your child with a range of issues which affect them and help us prevent further problems.

Initial assessment

During the initial assessment, the therapist will gather information about the issues and your child's background. This will help us reach an understanding of what brought your child to therapy, and work out the best ways to help resolve these problems and reduce any negative effects they are having.

You and the therapist will develop a shared understanding of the problems you want to work with and an agreed plan of care. The type and amount of input will vary, depending on the child's individual needs and our ability to help. This plan will be agreed at the end of your assessment.

Treatments

Any treatment recommendations will be discussed fully with you at the end of the first assessment.

We work closely with all agencies your child is involved with, so that the recommendations can be embedded into the child's life. If they are at school or nursery or community home, we may see your child there for a review of their care. This may follow an episode of care or when they have reached the target set for them. If this happens, a letter will be sent out to you letting you know the date and inviting you to attend if you wish. On these visits, your child may not necessarily be seen; the purpose of the visit may be to catch up with the staff at the sitting, check on the child's progress or treatment plan, or even observe the child in class.

'Do I have a problem? I don't want to do anything about it.'

---

4 DiClemente CC, Prochaska JO. Toward a comprehensive, transtheoretical model of change: stages of change and addictive behaviors. In: Miller WR, Heather N, editors. *Treating Addictive Behaviors*. 2nd ed. Plenum Press; 1998. pp. 3–24. Prochaska JO, Norcross JC, DiClemente CC. *Change for Good*. Quill; 2002.

Even if your child's needs are of significant impact, we may suggest that we wait before recommending treatment. Some children have difficulties that we know will resolve in time without help. Other, often older, children may not yet be willing or ready to put in the necessary time and effort. If this happens, we have to wait until the child is aware that they have a difficulty, and is motivated enough to want to put the work in. This may not happen for some months, and if this is the case, we always recommend that you contact us when the child herself (not you or school!) requests help through saying something like:

> 'I am getting some help and am practising daily.'

> Or 'I know I have a problem and am struggling.'

End of therapy

> 'I've learnt how to help myself and practise whenever I walk to the bus.'

> 'I do not have the problem any more.'

> 'I can do this most of the time in everyday life.'

> 'I may still have difficulty, but is no longer a problem for me.'

When the therapy ends, it is time to celebrate your child's achievements. She will have worked hard over a period of time, and rightly can be proud of the way her difficulties are resolving, or she learning to cope with her difficulties. The point at which therapy stops may not necessarily be when the issues are fully resolved, but when the child, or those close, to her has learnt the techniques that enable her to employ the strategies taught, and so is able to continue making progress by herself.

It is hoped that at the end of therapy there will be some resolution to the problem or at least some way of understanding and coping with the difficulties in more satisfactory ways. Therapy should not be seen as a cure in the same way that is sometimes applied to other medical conditions. It is usual that people finish therapy with some aspects of their problems unresolved. The intended benefits may be an improvement of your child's symptoms, but may also lead to increased self-confidence and easier, more satisfying relationships with others. Other benefits may be related to the specific issues presenting.

We hope this information is helpful for us all to work together to help your child. If you have any questions, please do not hesitate to ask.

The key thing is to work collaboratively, and support people in their decision making by communicating and keeping them informed. The aim is to develop a shared understanding of the problem with the patient, or the child and her carers.

For this to happen successfully, you as the clinician need to take the following steps.

➤ Explain your role as a part of the clinical team you work within.

➤ Explain your specific clinical role. At this stage, 'signpost' what happens when your specific support is complete, and who the patient may approach for further or ongoing care – for example, a counselling service for personal support, the GP for umbrella care, or a patient group for ongoing support around complex disability. Explaining discharge does not necessarily mean that all the issues will have been resolved. What we hope for is a better understanding of the difficulties and a better ability to cope.

➤ Explain the treatment trajectory: will it be given in episodes, be complete after one session, be time limited or be ongoing through life?

➤ What will your input be? Consider your ability to help, without delivering false promise. How can you be most effective? A programme, supporting life skills? Who is best placed to deliver the care? Define the type of care to be delivered and explain it, whether it will be group or individual, delivered by a registrar or nurse.

THE SECOND STEP: PLANNING THE CARE THROUGH REFLECTIVE THINKING

Patients are now, quite rightly, encouraged to be co-partners in their care. And, as we have seen, for this to work, patients need good information so they can make their choices. This has been referenced recently in relation to cancer care, where there are perceived funding issues for people with a terminal illness. As we discussed above, a debate about where medical care realistically has limitations and limits is needed.[5]

As we know, is not just healthcare workers who raise concerns about healthcare rationing. Others too have a stake in the discussion: charities, family, the media. All too often, the debate becomes heated as people confer with the media assumption that the National Institute for Health and Care Excellence (NICE) is working against the patients' best interest and is only interested in saving money. There is a debate to be had, with very valid views on both sides, but for our purposes we need to consider again: given the funding reality, how can we best meet the needs of all our patients? Clinicians need to be seen to be working in an effective, evidence-based way, and while NICE is rarely seen as an impartial body, one of its aims is to work to make fair decisions to protect us from expensive drugs that may work against our ultimate well-being. NICE is an honest adjudicator, and we too need to develop the kind of advanced

---

5 McCartney M. *The Patient Paradox: why sexed up medicine is bad for your health*. Pinter & Martin Ltd; 2012.

clinical thinking that NICE demonstrates in order to be taken seriously as clinicians, and to help us in our difficult discussions with patients.

Difficult conversations are hard, and many clinicians fudge the issue by using budgetary constraints as the fall guy to protect themselves from being the bearer of bad news. It is difficult, but essential, for us as carers to acknowledge when we have nothing more to offer, and honestly and openly to justify our clinical decision and reasoning. Our job is made less easy when fellow professionals (who may be unaware of their colleagues' thought processes, discussions and plans) support patients in their demand for care.

Thoughtful care planning aims to empower patients and clients of all ages and remove any unnecessary dependency on services. It challenges some of our own preconceptions as carers, as it is way of working that encourages us to stop identifying the problems, and think instead about the difficulties the patient is having and the current impact of these. Trusts are developing protocols to encourage and support staff to manage patient expectations and to manage the patient journey explicitly and objectively. One way is through the development of care plans. Care planning is mandatory for every child for whom we have an active duty of care. It is essential to achieve the 2011 Care Quality Commission standards and will be audited by them.

Patient expectation has developed over years, beginning with a very paternalistic and autocratic delivery of medicine, which encouraged patient deference, dependency and powerlessness. Traditionally, we devolved power to medical personnel, especially doctors, and as a result they today enjoy an unparalleled degree of trust and respect from the public. The pros and cons of this have been recognised in current medical school teaching, where expert communication skills are taught, and today doctors are much more likely to empower their patients through involvement in their treatment process. However, history and culture dictates that there is a residue of expectation from patients regarding the NHS:

➤ that the NHS will give whatever is needed for as long as is needed
➤ the NHS can fix/cure everything
➤ cure is better than prevention
➤ help will be effortless for the patient
➤ help will be 'free' and 'given' freely
➤ healthcare is a right.

This thinking is being challenged. The NHS Constitution[6] acknowledges that the NHS does belong to the people, and it is comprehensive and free of charge,

6 Department of Health. *The NHS Constitution: the NHS belongs to us all.* Department of Health; 2010.

but it sets out the rights to which the public, patients and staff are entitled, including:

➤ access to NHS services is based on clinical need
➤ the NHS is committed to providing best value for taxpayers' money and the most effective fair and sustainable use of finite resources
➤ you have the right to drugs and treatments that have been recommended by NICE for use in the NHS, if your doctor says they are clinically appropriate for you.

Patients also have the right to:

➤ make choices about their care, and to information to support these choices
➤ be involved in discussions and decisions about their healthcare and to be given information to enable them to do this.

We now respect the need for the patient to be empowered and share the responsibility, not simply be in receipt of the care. If we consider that access to NHS services is based on clinical need, and that we are custodians of taxpayers' money, it makes sense that as clinicians and managers we need to make the most effective, fair and sustainable use of these finite resources. Patients do not have the right to any drugs and treatments – they need, first, to have been recommended (by NICE) and, secondly, to be considered clinically appropriate. So, in order to limit the impact of patient expectation, and to challenge our own clinical thinking, we must not continue working as we always have, but must ask ourselves a different set of questions that stretch our clinical thinking, as developed by Malcomess,[7] and others.

➤ What does the patient/client/carer want to be different and can this be achieved? Will this happen anyway without our help? *Why* are you helping? *Can* you help? Keep asking yourself *why*. If you cannot answer any of these, you should not be helping.
➤ Think about *whose* need is being met – the child's, the carers', the service's or yours? Your focus must be the child. Many of us work in the caring profession because we do care, but this care, although hugely important, must not cloud clinical judgement. A paediatric consultant[8] recently spoke of his dismay when one of his patients was taken abroad by her parents to take part in unproven medical treatment – alternative medicine – as the parents had said that they 'would never forgive themselves if' they had not tried. The child returned to the UK in a worsened clinical state, with new

7 Malcomess K. The Care Aims model. In: Anderson C, van der Gaag A, editors. *Speech and Language Therapy: issues in professional practice*. Whurr Publishers Ltd; 2005.
8 Michalski A. Great Ormond Street. Hard to watch the suffering children. *The Times*. 2012 May 9.

medical complications. This was not, Michalski pointed out, about parents forgiving themselves. It was about the best thing for their child.

It is in the patients' best interest to become a partner in the care. Ethically, patients cannot be forced to follow a lifestyle dictated by others. Patients as consumers have the right to make their own choices and the ability to act on them. It is well known now that in the management of long-term illness and disability, increased knowledge on the part of the patient leads to empowerment and greater control.[9] Expert Patients Programme self-management courses ask their patients to control their condition instead of letting it control them. These self-management courses provide tools and techniques to help people take charge of their health and manage their condition better on a daily basis. The courses offer the confidence, skills and knowledge to manage chronic health conditions such as arthritis, asthma, diabetes, epilepsy, heart disease and multiple sclerosis.

According to advocates of this health movement, the following are key tenets of patient empowerment.

For the patient:

➤ care is delivered as close as possible to the patient
➤ patients and their carers are empowered fully to understand their condition and its needs
➤ patient anxiety is reduced
➤ holistic care is advocated and broader issues are addressed – courses include topics such as dealing with pain, extreme tiredness, coping with feelings of depression, relaxation techniques, exercise, healthy eating, communicating with family, friends and healthcare professionals, and planning for the future.

For the health service provider:

➤ expensive resources are freed up to research and develop services to meet unmet need; care can be devolved to trained and educated carers with just as much, if not more, benefit
➤ preventive medicine requires patient empowerment for it to be effective
➤ clinically, it has been shown that patient empowerment is an effective approach to address the psychosocial aspects of living with long-term conditions such as diabetes, degenerative neurological disease, stroke, pain management
➤ research shows it is conducive to improving some medical control over the condition (*see* below)

---

9 Department of Health. *The Expert Patient: a new approach to chronic disease management for the 21st century*. Department of Health; 2002. Donaldson L. Expert patients usher in a new era of opportunity in the NHS. *BMJ*. 2003; **329**: 1279.

➤ as clinicians, we work hard to empower our patients and carers through education and support programmes – treatment and care can be embedded in the patient's life, 24 hours a day, once they understand the supporting strategies.

Two clinical examples below, one from the acute sector and one from primary care, indicate the clinical benefits of devolving care as close as possible to the patient. They also help to demonstrate how one to one, clinically delivered care may not be the best care model, and show how important it is for us clinicians to 'sell' our clinical reasoning honestly, clearly and assertively.

The acute model

A 2007 US randomised, weight-listed control group trial was set to determine whether participation in a patient empowerment programme would result in improved psychosocial self-efficacy and attitudes toward diabetes, as well as a reduction in blood glucose levels. Results showed that:

➤ the intervention group showed gains over the control group on four of the eight self-efficacy subscales and two of the five diabetes attitude subscales

➤ the intervention group showed a significant reduction in glycated haemoglobin levels

➤ within groups, analysis of data from all programme participants showed sustained improvements in all of the self-efficacy areas and two of the five diabetes attitude subscales and a modest improvement in blood glucose levels.

The study indicated that patient empowerment is an effective approach to developing educational interventions for addressing the psychosocial aspects of living with diabetes. Furthermore, patient empowerment is conducive to improving blood glucose control.

The community model: consultative working

Since consultative working has been the norm for paediatric community thera-pists, we have seen the enormous benefits to our client group in embedding children's care in their own environment, freeing us up for training the care and support staff and working on the best ways to support those with long-term need. Children with specific speech/language impairment, for example, will have long-term, impacted communication needs. Many of these children will have entrenched communication difficulties throughout their life, despite one to one therapy input. Once these children reach adolescence, clinical reasoning dictates that any care plan must have these long-term needs at its heart.

With this in mind, we aim at secondary school level to gather information about the child's current needs and any current and outstanding issues, influences and impacts that will indicate the best ways to work with. The aim is to develop a shared understanding and an agreed plan of care. The type and amount of input will depend on a child's individual needs and motivation and our ability to help.

We work closely with schools and parents, so that the work can be embedded into the child's life. We aim for any strategies to be applied 24 hours a day and supported and understood by friends and family. Thus, for children with language difficulties in secondary school, the first focus is on training and supporting the school staff so that they understand the best ways to modify the curriculum to allow the child to access it better. The second focus is providing a programme with the aim that school will embed the ideas within its delivery and also deliver targeted and individualised help. The clinical reasoning behind this is a follows.

1   Adolescents – and their teachers – often state a preference for in-class working, as children of this age do not like to be seen as 'different' when removed from their peer group for programme delivery.

2   All work must have a functional bias. Programme ideas may be both direct (e.g. enhancing vocabulary) and indirect (e.g. assertiveness training). Programmes must be seen as meaningful to the child: they can see the application and benefits clearly, such as improving life skill.

3   At this stage, young adolescents have other strong focuses: academic, social, etc., so time and motivation for 'direct' work is low.

4   There is strong evidence for consultative working from many sources. If teachers can adapt the way they work – using communication-friendly strategies, for example – all children benefit, as individual learning styles are recognised and catered for. The language and learning impaired need material presented visually, kinaesthetically, simplified and shortened. This will need to be delivered in every contact with the child to allow them to access the curriculum.

5   Current research suggests that programmes can be delivered equally well by trained staff.[10] The aim of any therapy programme for this diagnostic category is that there will be some resolution to the problem, or at or at least some way of understanding and coping with the difficulties in more satisfactory ways. The intended benefits may be an improvement of the

10 Cirrin FM, Schooling TL, Nelson NW, *et al.* Evidence-based systematic review: effects of different service delivery models on communication outcomes for elementary school-age children. *Language, Speech, and Hearing Services in Schools.* 2010; **41**(3): 233–64.

symptoms, but will also include increased self-confidence and easier, more satisfying relationships with others. Other benefits may be related to the specific issues presenting.

The Cirrin study conducted an evidence-based systematic review of peer-reviewed articles from the last 30 years on the effect of different service delivery models on speech-language intervention outcomes for elementary school-age students. Structured review procedures were used to select and evaluate data-based studies that used experimental designs of the following types: randomised clinical trial, non-randomised comparison study and single-subject design study. The results, while acknowledging the need for further expanded research, indicated that classroom-based direct services are at least as effective as pull-out intervention for some intervention goals, and that highly trained speech-language pathology assistants, using manuals prepared by speech-language pathologists to guide intervention, can provide effective services for some children with language problems.

THE THIRD STEP: COMMUNICATING UNWANTED NEWS

As we have seen, patients need to be empowered, and part of this empowerment is being given good information so that they can make their choices. This has been referenced recently in relation to cancer care, where there is a debate about the impact of end of life care on patients and their families.[11] We are beginning to support some terminally ill patients in their understanding that they may be better off forgoing certain treatments that could provide 'false hope' in the final weeks of their lives. Not every patient has this view, nor every carer. But in order that we are seen as equal partners in the patients' care, we have to listen to those needs and wants, and give them our due consideration. Writing in the *Lancet Oncology* journal, academics led by Professor Richard Sullivan at King's College London have said the medical profession has a tendency to 'over-diagnose, over-treat and overpromise'. They are opening the debate that in sparing people futile and expensive end of life treatments, the health service could save money and may actually improve care:

> 'If we could accurately predict when further disease-directed therapy would be futile, we clearly would want to spare the patient the toxicity and false hope associated with such treatment, as well as the expense.'[12]

---

11 McCartney, note 5 above.
12 Sullivan R, Peppercorn J, Sikora K, *et al*. Delivering affordable cancer care in high-income countries. *Lancet Oncol*. 2011; **12**: 933–80.

This view is considered and thoughtful, and the result of advanced reflective thinking. The clinicians here are thinking holistically and very carefully about the impact of the disease and treatment, and the spiritual, emotional and psychological needs of the patient as well as their health needs. In order to get to this place, we need to broaden our understanding of the limits of what we can deliver, and be able to communicate this kindly, fairly and compassionately to our patients. For this we need to make ourselves as aware as we can abut the patient's background, their thinking, and their intellectual and emotional abilities to take in new, and difficult, information.

It is more than hard to communicate the very worst news. The timing is never great for the patient or for the clinician. We never know exactly what we are talking into: the very particular and special life circumstances of our patients. The clinical circumstances may not be great either: as a clinician you may be rushed, your clinic overbooked, your support staff may not be to hand, the patient may present without a relative or carer. The news has to be delivered fast, so clinically things can move to the next stage, but perhaps fast is not what the patient can cope with. There are many horror stories that we try to avoid: relatives that are told something different from the patient, people who are given the wrong information, people who have bald facts thrust on them clumsily by untrained personnel. All this has to be avoided. In an ideal world, we check out what people want to know before delivery. In an ideal world, we know the answers too. If we give a definitive diagnosis and prognosis, we have to be 100% certain – and it is rare that either can be predicted with that level of accuracy.

There may be an argument for not being prescriptive about predictions of morbidity and mortality with the life-limited patient and his or her relatives. Unless we are 100% certain, anything else said is just within the realms of probability, given that life is predictably uncertain and every one of us is our own unique mix of genetic inheritance and disease, with differing environmental, social, psychological impacts. The wife who was told her husband had 'probably' six months to live – a safe, measured, communication – was furious when he lived for 10 months. Furious because she had heard six months, prepared herself for six months, planned for six months. She would not have pushed him to do so much had she known they had 'all that extra time'. The second wife, told the same 'probable' six months, but whose husband died at three months, felt cheated. The death came too soon: unprepared, she had not allowed time for X, Y, Z that she had planned for the last months.

Maybe we are safer talking in generalities. We are not going to get it right because we do not know. But if we are fortunate enough to have cared for the patient throughout, we are going to have given him and his family all the right information at the very beginning of their journey, so these last signposts will not be foreign to them. We will know about the effects of prediction on cancer patients (there is some, anecdotal, evidence that if mortality dates are predicted and told to the patient they duly live to those dates). Better to check out how much information the patient wanted at diagnosis; discuss prognosis (in loose terms: 'People with this disease can live five, maybe 15 years … a normal lifespan, if we work hard together to control it …'), and acknowledge the difficulties of living with uncertainty. Offer all the levels of support needed, both practical ('This is how you can clean the PICC line.') and emotional ('If you need any extra emotional support we have counsellors on hand.'). Patients and their relatives need honesty, to be given the same information, openly and clearly, with the proviso that the quality and quantity of this information needs very careful handling.

For the patient, a common reaction to chronic uncertainty is the belief that real life will begin only when the period of uncertainty is over. With any prognosis open to doubt, a life that was once certain becomes a temporary condition, to be suffered not lived. Once the period of uncertainty begins to announce itself as the only certainty, life can become real again, even though utterly transformed.[13] If the uncertainty is accepted and not resisted, life is then lived again once more. A central tenet of the psychological therapist's work with patients with a life-limiting illness is bringing them to understand this level of uncertainty – that life, and when we die, is not certain for any of us.[14] Within this, there needs to be recognition that for most people a normal level of uncertainly is unknown; all life is untried and early death unlikely. The patient with a life-limiting condition has an enhanced level of uncertainty thrust upon them, a new awareness of mortality, and it will take time for them to come to terms with the new terms of their life. But by making counsellors and psychological therapists part of the oncology team, in particular, we may help encourage our patients to return to themselves and be defined not just by their disease, but by themselves.

Awareness of culture and personalities

Without a broad understanding and acknowledgement of how people become how they are, any communication with the patient or carer will be doomed. At the root of excellent interpersonal communication skills is the recognition that your communication partner is another human being with a wholly different take on the world to yours. As someone wise once said: 'Everyone believes in something people would rather they didn't.' And life would be much easier if we were all the same, but, sadly, most conflict arises when this assumption is made.

---

13 Mangusto S. The poet at bay. *New York Review*. 2011 Nov 26.
14 *See* www.cci.health.wa.gov.au/ (accessed April 2013).

Some of the things we need to be aware of when communicating any news, but particularly bad news, is the tendency for poor understanding on the part of the clinician about the exact personal history and personality of the patient, and poor understanding about the continuum of emotional health. Different strategies work to support people at different stages: the anxious patient has very different presentation and coping strategies to the one with a significant health phobia; the mildly anxious patient may be able to focus and take in what is being said; someone in an acutely anxious state may appear to be listening and understanding, but their fear response may mean that they are not able to be 'present' in the same way.

If the circumstances or behaviours of your client are particularly challenging, re-read Section 2. Otherwise, carry the awareness that delivering bad news is always an unhappy and complex task. Here are some ideas on how and how not to do it.

How not to do it

If in doubt, wait. If you are feeling vulnerable, tired or distracted: wait. Wait until you can give your full attention. Listen. Hear. Collect your thoughts, avoid rushing. Do not avoid eye contact and do not look at your computer or equipment. Sit at the same level as the patient. Be honest, but with care. Do not say anything that is un-thought out, overly clinical or patently unsympathetic, such as 'We've reached the end of the line', 'We are all going to die sometime', 'Any more treatment will be futile', 'There is no more (effective) treatment' (unless you add a rider: 'There may be no more effective clinical treatment but we can offer X, Y and Z …'). Any of these thoughtless comments would be crass, would undermine each patient's personal experience, and would demote their experience.

How to do it

Check out 'where' the patient is: do not assume. Your aim is to find out more about the patient and what they want: be assertive, clear and honest in your communication. The key thing is honesty. Work from a position of open curiosity: Ask, Ask and Ask.

➤ 'How do you feel about X?'
➤ 'What would you say to Y?'
➤ 'Who would you like to be involved with this?'
➤ 'When would you prefer B?'
➤ 'Where would you prefer C?'
➤ 'Tell me your feelings about A …'

Your aim is to find out more about the patient and what they want: be assertive, clear and honest in your communication.

Even if people in our care cannot be 'cured', it does not mean that we cannot give them valuable treatment, care and support. Our aim is to work with what will, at its heart, be a conflicted situation. The conflict arises from a mismatch of expectation, of hope, of dreams. Clinicians have a duty to manage this assertively: calmly, kindly, honestly and with compassion.

Work out what underlies the patient's response. Are they hurt, angry, anxious, terrified? We know that conflicts are nearly always caused by people having different points of view, or by people trying to achieve what they want at the expense of others. Understanding the nature and causes of the conflict and being able to use a wide range of approaches to prevent and resolve conflict are essential skills. Review some of the strategies mentioned in this book for resolving conflict, and consider especially that we can help to *prevent* conflicts by recognising and accepting differences between individuals in terms of values, perceptions, expectations and needs, and being honest with oneself and with others. We need to allocate sufficient time and energy really to get to know the patient so that we understand their values, beliefs, etc. This can be especially problematic in the current climate, where patients are not always reviewed by the same clinician, and patient contact sessions are often limited. We must not automatically assume we are right and they are wrong, and must not feel defensive if others disagree with us. This will help to enable people to express their feelings.

Successful conflict resolution is based on an accurate and thorough understanding of the difficulty presenting. Elsewhere in the book, we have talked about the broad approaches that can be taken for successful conflict resolution; each should match the particular circumstances presenting. In this instance, there is no room for clinicians to deny, suppress or withdraw information. They must collaborate together to reach an emotional compromise with their patient. Here, resolution occurs when each party gives something up in order to meet half way. We want the patient to be involved: 'I feel it is time to stop this particular treatment, as it is … causing you such distress/doesn't seem to be working in the way we want/not having the expected outcome/…, but I want you to be happy with my decision so shall I give you a few weeks to consider what we have said and if I don't hear from you …' This approach can be satisfactory if both parties have sufficient room to alter their positions, even though overall commitment to the 'agreed upon' solution may be in doubt. When collaborating in this way, individual differences are recognised, and the aim is for consensus, so both participants feel that they have won. If we make time for this approach, we will achieve a desired outcome.

The best way of dealing with breaking bad news is to be proactive, so that we both minimise the shock and prepare ahead for a resolution. We can do this by keeping patients informed, through using excellent interpersonal communication skills (be welcoming, attentive, helpful, and keep negative opinions to ourselves) and giving patients copies of correspondence relating to them, with a glossary of medical abbreviations and terms. We can demonstrate respect for the patient in all our dealings with them, discuss any relevant policies and procedures in advance (e.g. 'We anticipate the treatment cycle will be X, and if all goes well Y …') and make certain that records are available when the patient consults – we do not want to antagonise further. Through auditing complaints and plaudits, categorising the reason for a failure and naming those responsible, we can collectively discuss and implement ways to solve the problem.

According to a millennium report from the General Medical Services,[15] the most common patient complaints are with poor communication: inappropriate or ineffective care management or the complainer having some association with bereavement, grief or delayed/ailed diagnosis. Common negative patient experiences are usually due to poor communication: with professionals or, within the system, variations in service provision, poor information, lack of understanding/acknowledgement of the real emotional issues affecting the patient and carers, and bureaucracy and hierarchies benefiting the system not the patients. This can be avoided by having at the root of all people contact excellent communication. Immediately communicate bad news – do not cause further delay or anguish. Discussions must be real and important, otherwise they will be perceived as a standard, and impersonal, business response. Set the scene first, explaining why you are calling the patient in general terms. Use the time to refer to any previous discussions around the subject, and acknowledge any anxiety and anticipate any problems ('This all must have been very difficult for you'). Give the clinical details, as simply, clearly and concisely as you can, and finish with what you now propose for the future, allowing the listener time to absorb the information and react.

When communicating unwelcome news, we must anticipate that we will cause deep distress. We must communicate honestly and without defence: patients and relatives have a right to know – it is them, or their loved ones, we are discussing. Because of this we need to share with empathy: think about body language, eye contact and language use.

Never use euphemisms – they are unclear communication and misunderstandings will happen. Be clear, direct and honest: look at the person directly, sitting close to them.

It may be useful to reinforce the news by reading, or taping, any related correspondence together – people forget when distressed. Keep checking that you have been understood. Make use of trained counsellors to supervise and debrief – not other doctors, unless they have received special training. We

---

15 Green DR, Head of Risk Management, General Medical Services. The rising tide of complaints. *Pulse*. 2000 Dec 15.

should be very careful about using humour and flippancy to defend ourselves against any feelings generated – we are not the ones that need the defences.

We should anticipate strong emotional reactions in situations where they are likely to be provoked, and when this happens it is important that we acknowledge the situation and allow the patient space to talk through their feelings before discussing any priorities or offering alternatives. If anger emerges, signal your own openness to the feelings[16] by relaxing: breathe deeply to signal non-aggression. Use sympathetic/empathetic touch, stand or sit at slight angle, make good personal space. Keep your face in tune: if you smile inappropriately it will be read as a smirk. Be aware of gender, culture and ethnicity differences. Discuss differences openly to learn more, interpret correctly and react appropriately (e.g. in some cultures direct eye contact with a superior is seen as rude). Try to elicit any feelings underlying the anger, such as hopelessness, despair, chronic pain. Actively listen and check understanding, and attend throughout by making good eye contact and leaning forward with arms unfolded. Do not interrupt – let them tell the story: narratives help diffuse the big emotions.

The angry, defensive patient

Avoid provoking an angry reaction. If you present as indifferent or try to be over-controlling, or blame, judge or misinform, you will rightly trigger defensive behaviour. In these circumstances, it is even more important to create and maintain a positive atmosphere by listening, remaining calm and centred, detached from the personality and focused on the facts rather than the position. Look for common ground and agree that disagreements can coexist. Aim for win-win.

If the patient leaves the room before you have a chance to continue, use reflective learning techniques to analyse the consultation: is there anything you could have done differently? Act quickly to get back in control, be positive and try to retrieve the patient yourself. Invite him to sit down – it is harder to be angry if you are both sitting.

Not all patients will react to bad news with anger or sadness. When people are worried or panicky, their intellect will shut down and they will react in more extreme ways. Physiologically, anxiety arouses the sympathetic nervous system, which in turn makes the amygdala more responsive to apparent threats and sensitises us to traces of past experiences, shaded with residues of fear. This intensifies trait anxiety: ongoing anxiety regardless of the situation. Meanwhile, frequent sympathetic nervous system activation wears down the hippocampus, vital for forming explicit memories – a clear record of what actually happens. Hence it is a bad combination for the amygdala to be over-sensitised while

---

16 Braithwaite R. Anger management. *Community Care.* 1999 Sep 16–22.

the hippocampus is compromised: more distorted and painful experiences are recorded in implicit memory, without any accurate explicit memory of them.[17] Most of us can remain reasonable and considerate most of the time, but (particularly if our personal history dictates) we break under certain circumstances. People who are already vulnerable need particularly careful handling. The frightened patient needs privacy, an acknowledgement of their distress and very sympathetic handling, with competent, firm reassurance. As we have seen, in people with extreme anxiety, a fear response kicks in, reducing their ability to engage cognitively or intellectually. If this is the case, or if your patient needs support to be competent, or has language difficulties, he or she will need you to take charge, so begin by clarifying essential details such as their age, address, type/site of pain. Give any details non-verbally, kindly and compassionately, and avoid spelling out rules. Support information with diagrams, symbols and gestures. If your patient loses all emotional control, do take time and wait a minute before offering sympathy or intervening, which might escalate the situation. Contain the feelings for the patient: 'Let's take a moment to collect our thoughts', and show your concern with the sympathetic use of body language.

The insecure patient

People who behave reactively are responding to external influences in an uncontrolled way, reactions that can be related to insecurity, unmet needs and fear,[18] so these feelings can be negated by asking: 'How secure do you feel here?', 'Are you getting what you need from us?', 'What are you scared of?' Aim instead to think carefully: respond, do not react, and look instead for a win-win outcome.

If we have a good self-image and self-esteem, we are able to think kindly of ourselves: 'I am someone who is thoughtful, caring, who has integrity.' Good self-esteem helps us to behave assertively in difficult situations: we respect the needs of others and ourselves; we care enough to have the courage to connect. We have awareness of, and commitment to, what we are doing. We have enough of ourselves to behave with humility. Not everyone is able to do this. If focussed on ego we would behave arrogantly, greedily, competitively and in a self-focussed way.

➤ Do not greet all patient suggestions with a reason why it will not work, or cannot be done: respond with a positive or alternative suggestion.
➤ Be assertive: if the patient asks for something unreasonable, respond reasonably: 'I won't be able to do that, at the moment this other treatment takes priority.'

---

17 Hanson R, Mendius R. *Buddha's Brain: the practical neuroscience of happiness, love and wisdom.* New Harbinger Publications; 2009.
18 Braithwaite, note 16 above.

➤ Make yourself aware of the effect of your behaviour on other people.
➤ Seek out constructive criticism. Ask for feedback, and be prepared for frankness!
➤ Mind your own ego.
➤ Respect people and other approaches.
➤ Focus on commonalities rather than differences.
➤ Avoid gender-biased attitudes, categorising and generalising.
➤ Describe instead of interpreting.
➤ What is your intention in the interaction? Are you operating according to your principles or in response to someone else's?

Conflict will always occur when there is miscommunication, conflict between personality types, differing values, perceptions and opposing objectives. Stress occurs when our perception colours an event that has triggered us emotionally. We are more likely to react angrily if stressed. In both instances, we need to find the common ground. However difficult any discussions are going to be perceived, remember that conflict can be positive when it helps to open up an issue, and this results in problems being solved. Naturally, those that are likely to result in positive outcomes support us to try the same technique again. And negative-outcome conflicts have to be either prevented or reflected on, and acknowledged and resolved in a positive manner.

KEY POINTS

➤ There are some groups of patients for whom any news is going to be perceived as additionally threatening, because of their own life story, medical history or mental health issues. So there are times when the need to be intuitive, empathic and assertive – using clear, honest and open communications – is courageous and crucial.
➤ As humans, we struggle to face the unknown: we like to feel we are in control of our destinies, and have yet to confront fully the processes of managing uncertainty, illness, difficulty, disability, our own deaths.
➤ Public institutions contain what is disowned by the rest of society: in this way, they become an arena for the contestability of public concerns .This may help to explain the outrage when advanced medical technologies cannot be made available to all, or the tendency to feel duped when interventions fail.
➤ While we expect treatment always to end in cure and medicine to be delivered without patient engagement or effort, the NHS will always be raised on a dais of our own making.
➤ To limit the impact of patient expectation and challenge our own clinical thinking, stop identifying the problems and think instead about the *need* and *impact.*

➤ Work collaboratively. Patients need good, unbiased, well-delivered information about their choices – about the treatment, its limits and their own responsibilities – so expectations are not raised unnecessarily. Inform about roles, the treatment trajectory, and any limitations or limits of the care you provide.

➤ A rationing debate is called for, with very valid views on both sides, but for our purposes we need to consider again: given the funding reality, how can we best meet the needs of all our patients?

➤ History and culture dictates a residue of expectation from patients regarding the NHS. This thinking is being challenged, to inform the public that access to NHS services must be based only on clinical need. Within this, we also think holistically, considering the spiritual, emotional and psychological needs of the patient as well as their health needs. Even if people in our care cannot be 'cured', it does not mean that we cannot give them valuable treatment, care and support. Our aim is to work with what will, at its heart, be a conflicted situation. The conflict arises from a mismatch of expectation, of hope, of dreams. Clinicians have a duty to manage this assertively: calmly, kindly, honestly and with compassion. Collaborate together to reach an emotional compromise.

➤ It is in the patient's best interest to become a partner in the care. In the management of long-term illness and disability, increased knowledge on the part of the patient leads to empowerment and greater control. For the NHS, expensive resources are freed up.

➤ Without a broad understanding and acknowledgement of how people become how they are, any communication with the patient or carer will be doomed. Different strategies work to support people at different stages.

➤ If you have to deliver bad news, but are feeling vulnerable, tired or distracted, wait. Be honest, but with care. Check out 'where' the patient is; do not assume. Work from a position of open curiosity: Ask, Ask and Ask. Your aim is to find out more about the patient and what they want.

➤ We should anticipate strong emotional reactions in situations where they are likely to be provoked. Do not interrupt, let people tell their story: narratives help diffuse the big emotions. Work out what underlies the patient's response: are they hurt, angry, anxious, terrified?

➤ When people are worried or panicky, their intellect will shut down and they will react in more extreme ways.

➤ Work on developing your own *self-esteem* as this helps you to behave assertively in difficult situations: respecting the needs of others and yourself, caring enough to have the courage to connect, and having awareness of, and commitment to, what you are doing. If focussed on *ego* we behave arrogantly, greedily, competitively.

FURTHER READING

Kurtz S, Silverman J, Draper A. *Teaching and Learning Communication Skills in Medicine.* 2nd revised ed. Radcliffe Publishing; 2004.

Tate P. *The Doctor's Communication Handbook.* 6th revised ed. Radcliffe Publishing; 2009.

Pendleton D, Schofield T, Tate P, *et al. The New Consultation: developing doctor-patient communication.* 2nd revised ed. Oxford University Press; 2003.

CHAPTER 14

Boundaries in clinical work

'Boundaries: "A line that marks the limits of an area; a dividing line; a limit of a subject or sphere of activity."'[1]

Online dictionary definition

In this concluding chapter of the section, we look at what working within boundaries means for us as clinicians, and how we make use of boundaries in assertiveness. To be assertive, one has to hold a boundary, hold the line. It is always a risk to be honest, clear and unambiguous: the risk of possibly not being liked, rejection at worst. We need to remember that saying 'no' does not always mean being unkind: the consequences of 'kindness' can be far worse and far reaching. Here we take a look at some clinical moral and ethical dilemmas, situations where boundaries have been breached, and consider the consequences, good and bad. There are never clear-cut solutions to these kinds of dilemmas – there can never be absolute resolution in life – but they are offered here to encourage readers to think through what they might have done, and what the healthiest solution may be.

We have seen how many of our clients will try to make us responsible for their behaviour, by making us responsible for all the decision making and work in managing their care. Historically, this has been so. But medicine is no longer paternalistic. Ultimately, the illness or presenting difficulty does not belong to the doctors, nor the parents/carers: it belongs to the patient. We know now that we need to empower people so they can make their recovery a joint venture. In developing a boundary, we tell them: 'This is yours, and this is mine'; we tell them what they, and we, are responsible for. There are deeper reasons for us to develop clinical boundaries: we need our patients and clients to trust us, so we need to behave in ways that make us transparently trustworthy.

This is never easy. We have seen that our own behaviour is often motivated by trying to appoint someone else – a boss, partner, colleague – to be responsible for our problems. It can be challenging to take responsibility, so in an attempt to reduce the pain of taking responsibility, we often take the easy route, giving

---

1 *Oxford Dictionary of English.* 2nd revised ed. Oxford University Press; 2010.

241

away our power. To regain that power, and to behave assertively, we need to be seen to act in ways that demonstrate we are empowered to accept any consequences of our decisions. The purpose of having boundaries as a clinician is to protect and take care of ourselves, in order to give the best service we can without being contaminated with our own issues, and also to set the limits that help support others to trust us. It is impossible to have a healthy relationship with anyone if they have no boundaries, as they are not communicating directly and honestly. Patients need us to hold the boundary so they can trust what we say is real. For some clients, it is crucial to know that their practitioner will act within a defined frame. For others, it is equally crucial that we can be seen to be flexible so that trust is established not on predictability but authenticity.[2]

In our ongoing work with clients, we also need to consider the demands of practice, legislation, registration and the recognition of our competencies. To practise safely we do need to be explicitly educated about boundaries and ethics. There is a fine line between practising defensively and practising safely. The concept of boundaries is coded in legal structures, and sometimes can force many of us into defensive practice, not working in ways that give clients the best clinical environment for their needs, but with the aim to avoid vulnerability to misconduct hearings. This is the core stuff of risk management: if we can demonstrate that we self-monitor, reflect, question, consider and, where necessary, seek support for our decision making (through accurate note keeping, supervision records, etc.), we are much better placed. Our clients/patients are not dangers to be negotiated, but people with whom we have a developing relationship.[3] We can afford to relax, provided we manage the risk. A balance has to be sought.

The chapter aims to guide, not to prescribe. Hopefully, it will help you think. The aim is to develop your understanding of how and why you respond in difficult situations, with people with difficult or demanding behaviour, and to give you some ideas of better, healthier ways of responding. We also look briefly at the developing concept of 'appropriate clinical boundaries'. Practitioners need to find ways of working that are based on giving the patient the best therapy, best suited to them, rather than being forced to work defensively, in ways to avoid vulnerability to criticism or disciplinary hearings.

As clinicians, we follow some fundamental ground rules when we work, which help keep people, safe. We recognise the importance of setting ground rules such as seeing people at a set time, in a clinical environment, with no gifts being accepted. We may add the importance of notifying clients of any protocol for non-attendance, not setting up inappropriate personal relationships with clients, etc. There is an absolute need strictly to adhere to these rules. These

2   Totton N. Boundaries and boundlessness. *Therapy Today*. 2010; **21**(8): 11–15.
3   Ibid.

national and local arrangements seem to match the unconscious need of every client for safety, clarity and understanding.[4]

Instinctively, we know that adherence to boundaries keeps us as clinicians safe too. Slack working always leads practitioners into vulnerable areas: misunderstanding, insufficient self-monitoring or misbehaviour. However, in the extreme, working defensively leads us to neither liking nor trusting those we work with. On one level, the threat is to the practitioner's standing, should a complaint be made, but the real threat is to the practitioner's insecure self-image and self-esteem. We become our worst internal critic. A happy medium needs to be found. We need to retain some sense of flexibility, perhaps with the human qualities of attention, care and warmth, while maintaining a safe space for the client to work in. We need to stand firm and, to help us as practitioners feel safe, we need our managers to uphold any protocols by supporting us if a complaint is made, not deviating from the 'rules' and allowing the complainer different treatment.[5]

SETTING THE BOUNDARIES

First of all, we need to be clear about, and explain, our role with the patient: who we are and how we work. We may need to learn a 'script' that we feel comfortable delivering. People need information that helps them understand how we can best help them to be given clearly and succinctly. We need to:
➤ set the scene
➤ identify the input
➤ explain who else might be involved.

People feel comfortable when they understand our expectations of them, the boundaries we work within, what our expectations of them are. We set the scene through giving out literature before the appointment, and also by explaining our specific role and how this links with other professionals, if appropriate. Give clear guidance about the limits of your role in order to reduce overdependence – emotional support for the patient may best be met by another colleague: a child's school, the GP, psychological support services. Secondly, identify the input. Explain how and when treatment will be given. All at once? In episodes? Over what period of time? Is treatment appropriate right now? Check that the patient understands this. Explain that the type of input may vary, depending on their level of need and our ability to help. Discuss how can you be most effective, and, if you are not best placed to deliver the care, explain who will

---

4 Smith DL. *Hidden Conversations: introduction to communicative psychoanalysis*. Routledge; 1991. Johnson SH, Farber BA. The maintenance of boundaries in psychotherapeutic practice. *Psychotherapy*. 1996; **33**: 391–402.

5 Totton, note 2 above.

be. All this requires good, clear, honest and assertive talking. We may need to address difficult issues. We may need to explain that a discharge does not necessarily mean a cure or that all the issues will have been resolved. We may successfully complete treatment, or what we may hope for is that the patient has a better understanding of the difficulties and a better ability to cope.

ETHICAL DILEMMAS AND REFLECTIVE PRACTICE

As clinicians, we are endlessly developing our awareness of ethical practice in the broader context of morals and values, and are becoming more familiar with the frameworks for ethical decision making. Our examination here of some common ethical issues in clinical practice also raises questions about service management. For many clinicians, boundaries are fundamental to our practice, even if not in our conscious awareness: where it is not, work needs to be done to make it part of our conceptual framework. The scenarios below help us consider those factors which complicate ethical decision making.

After reading the following dilemmas, unpick them. Consider the perspective of the different people within the experience. Each perspective will be motivated by personal, professional and organisational interests. Withdrawing from the situation in this way encourages the practitioner to move from his or her own partial view to gain an overall view.

It may be useful to consider patient autonomy from this perspective: the professional will consider they have the client's best interests at heart and act accordingly. In this light, respect the safeguarding agenda and the patient's right to be self-determining – enable them to make their own decisions. This is a principal that many healthcare workers have difficulty with. We have our own ideas of virtue or duty, how we would or should conduct ourselves. We are carers, and as such often let our own emotions influence our thinking: we may become over-involved. Within this, we often impose our own values into the situation ('If it were me …'). The problem with this principle is that the patient is not you (or your mother/child), and imposing this value may be misguided, particularly in the light of consent. Consider who has the authority for making the decision: always consider and reconsider your own autonomy, authority and accountability for making and acting on decisions. You may have legitimate *authority* (having considered all the issues of patient consent), but you may also believe you have *autonomy* in a particular area. Check and reflect on this. You must consider any power factors: the power relationship set up in any patient/clinician relationship, with the power held by the professional.

➤ Has the decision been made in terms of what is best for the patient?
➤ Has it considered the patient's views?
➤ Or are you working with an inherent belief in terms of your power base and perhaps fear of sanction. Has the patient simply been compliant?

Having considered all these different perspectives, and how they might be resolved, use them to inform your thinking. There will be a wrong way, a right way and another way, which may also be wrong or right. Nothing is prescriptive.

To recap, the Mental Capacity Act 2005 states that every adult has the right to make his or her own decisions and must be assumed to have capacity to do so unless it is proved otherwise. A patient does not have to show that he or she has capacity. We have to show they do not. We must remember that people must be supported as much as possible to make a decision before anyone concludes that they cannot make their own decision, and that they have the right to make what others might regard as an unwise or eccentric decision. We must guard against the kinds of prejudicial assumptions that tend to be made based on the patient's age, health status, appearance or behaviour. It is common to find these assumptions: they should never form part of our assessments or decision making in mental capacity testing or otherwise. The Department of Health has issued a range of guidelines on consent;[6] all professional bodies have their own guidelines; and each NHS trust sets out standards and procedures to help professionals to comply with the guidelines. Our responsibilities are clear and unequivocal:

➤ always to act in the best interests of the patient
➤ to obtain consent before treatment or care
➤ to be mindful of your legal and professional accountability when obtaining consent
➤ accurately to record discussions and decisions relating to obtaining consent.

There is no room for woolly thinking here – people have a fundamental right to make their own decisions, whether we like it or not.

Boundaries are guidelines that are based on the basic principles of clinical codes of ethics. Many professions – counsellors, social workers, the voluntary sector – have a long and developed history of looking at this. Sectors within the NHS are beginning to develop their own frameworks, including informed consent, open discussion, consultation, supervision, documentation, utilitarianism (an action is right if it produces the greatest good for the greatest number)[7] and examination of personal motivation.[8]

---

6 Lachmann PJ. Symposium on consent and confidentiality: consent and confidentiality – where are the limits? An introduction. *J Med Ethics*. 2003; **29**(1): 2–3. *See* www.doh.gov.uk/government/publications/reference-guide-to-consent-for-examination-or-treatment-second-edition/ (accessed May 2013).
7 Reamer FG. *Ethical Dilemmas in Social Service*. 2nd ed. Columbia University Press; 1990.
8 Corey G, Corey MS, Callanan P. *Issues and Ethics in the Helping Professions*. Brooks/Cole Publishing Co.; 1998.

Corey and others[9] outline five principles on which therapeutic boundaries are based. I specifically draw the reader's attention to the current British Association for Counselling & Psychotherapy website,[10] which has an excellent section on accountability and ethics: follow the link to 'Ethical frameworks'. Here these are adapted and expanded to suit any working relationship of those in the caring professions.

Principles for therapeutic boundaries

Beneficence: a commitment to promoting the client's well-being
This means:
➤ always acting in the best interests of the client
➤ working strictly within one's limits of competence
➤ providing services on the basis of adequate training or experience.

Ensuring that these outcomes are achieved requires systematic monitoring of practice and outcomes, through commitment to updating practice by continuing professional development, supervision, research and systematic reflection to inform practice. As we have seen, the obligation to act in the best interests of a client may become paramount when working with clients whose capacity for autonomy is diminished because of immaturity, lack of understanding, extreme distress, serious disturbance or other significant personal constraints.

Non-maleficence: a commitment to avoiding harm to the client
This involves:
➤ avoiding sexual, financial, emotional or any other form of client exploitation
➤ avoiding incompetence or malpractice
➤ not providing services when unfit to do so due to illness or personal circumstances
➤ no allowance for 'reckless' behaviour; we have to be constantly aware whether our actions or behaviour, considered or unconsidered, harm or not
➤ not setting up a 'dual relationship',[11] said to arise when the practitioner has two or more kinds of relationship concurrently with a client, for example client and trainee, acquaintance and client, colleague and supervisee; the existence of a dual relationship with a client is rarely

---

9 Beauchamp TL, Childress JF. *Principles of Biomedical Ethics*. 4th ed. Oxford University Press; 1994.
10 www.bacp.co.uk (accessed May 2013).
11 Bader E. Dual relationships: legal and ethical trends. *Transactional Analysis*. 1994; **24**(1): 64–6.

neutral and can have a powerful beneficial or detrimental impact, which may not always be easily foreseeable, so practitioners are required:

- to consider the implications of entering into dual relationships with clients
- to avoid entering into relationships that are likely to be detrimental to clients
- to be readily accountable to clients and colleagues for any dual relationships that occur.

The practitioner has an ethical responsibility to mitigate any harm caused to a client, even when the harm is unavoidable or unintended. We also have a personal and professional responsibility to challenge, where appropriate, the incompetence or malpractice of others; and to contribute to any investigation concerning professional practice which falls below that of a reasonably competent practitioner and/or risks bringing discredit upon our profession.

Autonomy: recognition and respect for the client's right to be self-governing

This principle emphasises the importance of the client's commitment to participating in any treatment, and opposes the manipulation of those we care for against their will. To enable this we need to be seen to:

➤ ensure accuracy in any information given in advance of services offered
➤ inform the patient/client in advance of foreseeable conflicts of interest or as soon as possible after such conflicts become apparent
➤ engage in explicit contracting in advance of any commitment by the client
➤ protect privacy and confidentiality by ensuring adequately informed consent:
    - confidential information about clients may be shared within teams where the client has consented or knowingly accepted a service on this basis; and the disclosure enhances the quality of service available to clients or improves service delivery
    - make explicit the 'rules' of breaking confidentiality: exceptional circumstances may prevent the practitioner from seeking client consent to a breach of confidence due to the urgency and seriousness of the situation, for example, preventing the client causing serious harm to self or others. In such circumstances, the practitioner has an ethical responsibility to act in ways which balance the client's right to confidentiality against the need to communicate with others. Disclosures of confidential information should be conditional on the explicit, signed consent of the person concerned, for example, 'I will need to contact X if we feel you are thinking of harming yourself or others, or if I become aware of a safeguarding issue'. Client consent is the only safe and ethical way of resolving any dilemmas over confidentiality

- Practitioners should be willing to be accountable to their clients and to their profession for their management of confidentiality in general, and particularly for any disclosures made without their client's consent. This is a situation that needs repair immediately. Good records of existing policy and practice and of situations where the practitioner has breached confidentiality without client consent greatly assist ethical accountability.

Respecting clients' privacy and confidentiality are fundamental requirements for keeping trust and respecting client autonomy. Service managers set up systems that ensure protection of personally identifiable and sensitive information from unauthorised disclosure. Disclosure may be authorised by client consent or the law. Any such disclosures should be undertaken in ways that best protect the client's trust and respect client autonomy.

Justice: the fair and impartial treatment of all clients and the provision of adequate services
➤ Being just and fair to all patients/clients and respecting their human rights and dignity.
➤ Practitioners need to consider any legal requirements and ethical obligations, and remain alert to potential conflicts between these.

As we have seen in the previous chapter, justice in the distribution of services requires the ability to determine impartially the provision of services for those we care for and the allocation of services between them. A commitment to fairness requires the ability to appreciate differences between people and to be committed to equality of opportunity, avoiding discrimination against people or groups contrary to their legitimate personal or social characteristics. Practitioners have a duty to strive to ensure a fair provision of services, accessible and appropriate to the needs of potential patients and clients too.

Fidelity: honouring the trust placed in the practitioner
Being trustworthy is regarded as fundamental to understanding and resolving ethical issues. Practitioners who adopt this principle: act in accordance with the trust placed in them; regard confidentiality as an obligation arising from the client's trust; restrict any disclosure of confidential information about clients to furthering the purposes for which it was originally disclosed.

Self-respect: fostering the practitioner's self-knowledge and care for self
The principle of self-respect means that the practitioner appropriately applies all the above principles as entitlements for self. This includes:
➤ seeking help for oneself if the need arises

➤ utilising opportunities for personal development as required
➤ using supervision for appropriate personal and professional support and development
➤ seeking training and other opportunities for continuing professional development
➤ guarding against financial liabilities arising from work undertaken usually requires that appropriate insurance cover is obtained.

Those who ignore these needs are not being true to themselves, and are certainly not behaving responsibly, assertively and professionally. Practitioners who, consciously or unconsciously, passively or deliberately, avoids supervision, or training, or asking for help if needed, are avoiding their responsibilities to their patients and are running a very high risk. We have a responsibility to ensure we remain alert to our professionalism; there is no excuse for avoidant behaviour here.

Boundaries are a crucial aspect of any effective clinician/client/patient relationship. They set the structure for the relationship and provide a consistent framework for the treatment process.[12] Some boundary lines are clear. Most GPs would acknowledge that it is ethically problematic, for example, to accept a friend or close relative onto their list because the pre-existing relationship impairs objectivity and serves to undermine the professional relationship. While situations such as these are clearly problematic, outside of such elementary confines are numerous situations where the delineation of boundaries is less clear. We sometimes feel that these situations fall outside of the formal code of ethics and lie instead in an ambiguous grey area, whereas in fact all interactions we have with clients fall within this area: when we accept a gift from a patient, for example. What we are aiming for is something suited to the patient/clients' changing needs and circumstances: not rigid, inflexible boundaries/guidelines, nor too much flexibility so both parties become enmeshed and neither understands the boundary.

Clearly, it would be counterproductive to the therapeutic relationship if we were so formal in our exchanges that we no longer empathised with the patient or client. However, nor do we want to empathise with the client to the extent that we hug the client on meeting them, or pop in to visit unannounced at the client's home on our own way home from the office. This is the behaviour of a friend, not a working relationship. Hence, boundary violation has occurred.

Ambiguous boundaries often arise in clinical work with patients, but strict responsibilities do apply to health workers in relation to their duty to inform clients of the limitations on client confidentiality. Such information forms a large part of informed consent, and informed consent is a fundamental

---

12 Available at: www.counsellingconnection.com (accessed April 2013).

client right. We must ensure that services are delivered on the basis of the client's explicit consent. Reliance on implicit consent is more vulnerable to misunderstandings and is best avoided unless there are sound reasons for doing so. Overriding a client's known wishes or consent is a serious matter that requires commensurate justification. Practitioners should be prepared to be readily accountable to clients, colleagues and their professional body if they override a client's known wishes.

Boundary violations

Here are some examples of boundary violations. Consider each one. There are no automatic rights and wrongs here, no clear answers. Whatever you choose, it is likely you will be left with uncomfortable feelings because there is no resolution that will satisfy all parties: there are rarely black and white solutions to these matters. However, it is worth considering, in each situation:[13]

➤ your personal core values and beliefs
➤ how these values sit with the organisation you work for
➤ the manner and content of what is said, and what this might communicate to people who use our services
➤ what the moral and ethical implications are
➤ how our conversation/discourse affirms or undermines client autonomy
➤ what would engage/disengage the patient/clients.

Consider the challenges too:
➤ confidentiality
➤ responsibilities, boundaries, privacy
➤ respecting loyalties to patients, colleagues, carers
➤ assertive decision making
➤ consent
➤ cultural issues
➤ moral versus clinical duty.

Discuss with colleagues. In the light of your discussion, are the decisions you make effective, efficient and equitable?

> **Scenario 1**[14]
> Felicity had been seeing Paul, her physiotherapist, as an outpatient for six months as part of ongoing treatment following her road traffic accident, when she was rushed to hospital for emergency surgery. As she was extremely

---

13 Body R, McAllister L. *Ethics in Speech and Language Therapy*. Wiley-Blackwell; 2009.
14 Adapted from *Boundaries*. Available at: www.counsellingconnection.com (accessed April 2013).

stressed and upset on the phone when she rang to cancel the scheduled appointment, Paul visited her at the hospital the following day, as he was running a clinic there. Felicity was in horrific pain, and Paul sat in a chair beside her bed and took her hand when she held it out to him. Paul offered some words of comfort and, after ensuring that the family would be visiting Felicity soon, he left the hospital.

Felicity was aware that this was an exception to her usual physiotherapy sessions with Paul and assumed it would not be repeated. She told herself that his visit to the hospital simply meant that he cared for her and could appreciate the depth of her pain and vulnerability.

At the first outpatient session with Felicity after her discharge from hospital, Paul took the first few minutes of the session to discuss his visit to the hospital to ensure that Felicity understood fully its place in the context of the clinical relationship. Paul was beginning to wish he had not visited, and felt uncomfortable that his intentions may be misconstrued. He was reassured by Felicity's understanding of the situation and they let the matter drop.

Considerations Scenario 1

➤ Would you have visited Felicity at the hospital? If not, why not? In what circumstances?

➤ Whose emotions are evoked here? Whose need is being met?

➤ Do you feel there is a role for practitioners to make their own decision in a situation such as this?

➤ Do you consider Paul's manner to be professional?

➤ What compromise would you make, if at all?

➤ Do you feel that Paul violated known boundaries?

➤ Are your responses emotional or professional, and does it matter?

➤ Who could you plan to talk to about this?

➤ Was Paul's behaviour appropriate as a professional, in a professional setting? Where do the boundaries between friendship and professional behaviour lie here? Are these lines clear-cut?

Discussion Scenario 1

While most health professionals would not have visited Felicity at the hospital, arguing that it took the therapeutic relationship outside of the confines of the set appointments and that Paul's behaviour could have been misinterpreted by the client, many other practitioners believe that a decision must be based on the individual circumstances and the uniqueness of each relationship with each individual client. Again, given clinical autonomy, each practitioner should make their own judgement, but this must be able to be defended, in court if necessary, or at the very least to their line manager and supervisor.

There is a view that the professional manner in which Paul conducted himself during the hospital visit and later at the first counselling session allowed him to move the boundaries in all good conscience. He was not cavalier about his visit to the hospital; rather, he carefully thought out his decision, considering the ramifications and benefits for his patient.

Taking this view, his behaviour was appropriate as a professional, in a professional setting: he did not make the mistake of thinking his visit was equal to that of a friend and neither did he behave as a friend. Also, as soon as he was able, he spoke to the client to clarify the visit and remove any possibility of ambiguity or innuendo. Hopefully too, he kept accurate and contemporaneous notes to explain his decision making and remove any ambiguity. Ideally too, he would have thought it a good idea – as he was considering going outside the normal boundaries of behaviour – to consult his line manager or supervisor first, so as not to be seen to act independently and possibly impulsively.

For counsellors in particular, ethical dilemmas such as these arise frequently, as intense feelings can emerge in the sessions which can often challenge a counsellor's personal and professional boundaries. However, all healthcare practitioners need to understand and consider fully the serious effects of their own personal power, and how that can be misinterpreted by the client. When counsellors choose to be flexible regarding boundaries, they do so carefully, having taken into account the ramifications of their flexibility for their client: this is something we need to learn about. For many of us working in less intense circumstances, we do not have to face the exact scenario above. However, there are a many circumstances where, morally and ethically, boundaries may be challenged in our work.

Scenario 2

A family has five children, the eldest two of whom were both under the care of two professionals from the same team, an occupational therapist and a speech and language therapist. Poppy was under the care of Crista, the speech and language therapist, and Sasha was under the care of Monica, the occupational therapist. Each therapist was clear about their individualised and specialised work with the family. Neither therapist had spent time formally discussing the family with the other: pressures of time meant this was rarely possible. However, both therapists had, in passing, over coffee, shared some of their general anxieties about the parental attitudes and involvement.

All went well until one day Crista visited the school to see Poppy, and Poppy's father asked her during the consultation whether she felt the other therapist, Monica, was right in her decision making about Sasha: did Crista feel that Sasha needed to have a statement of special educational needs? Crista, aware that she did not know Sasha at all clinically, felt uncomfortable, yet felt pushed to give a response. She quickly came up with a guarded, fairly neutral professional opinion, an opinion she felt was general, honest and non-committal: she said that statement was not always needed, and that parents did definitely need to consent to the process.

What Crista did not realise, was that Monica was working hard behind the scenes with the school and associated professionals (including the safeguarding team) to support the family towards accepting a difficult diagnosis, and that part of this work was gradually getting them to accept a statement for Sasha so that she could begin to receive the level of care she needed. The sub-text, too, was to draw the parents into the process so that they would begin to accept the complexity of Sasha's diagnosis, understand fully how to best support her and implement some of the recommendations. Crista's comment that not all children required statements by law led the parents to refuse to accept the statementing procedure, thus negating the significant amount of work already done. The next day, Monica was contacted by the school to update her on what had happened.

Considerations Scenario 2

➤ Whose case is this? Who holds professional responsibility for the family?
➤ What do you think the consequences of this were?
➤ How do you think you would have handled the situation?
➤ Was a boundary broken, and, if so, whose boundary was it?
➤ Are the responses emotional or professional, and does it matter?
➤ Who would you plan to talk to about this?
➤ What compromises would you make?

Discussion Scenario 2

Monica was, predictably, angry when she heard the news. She felt that confidentiality had been broken, a professional boundary had been crossed; she felt that Crista had interfered in her own decision making and caseload management. She was angry with herself for not predicting that this would happen, given the unusual circumstances, and wished that, despite time pressures, she thought to suggest that she and Crista set aside time to discuss how they should both behave if this scenario occurred, as it was likely to do so.

Almost simultaneously, Monica was remembering with shame and embarrassment that during *her* first consultation with Sasha's father, he had asked her opinion about Poppy in the same way. On this occasion, during the discussions around consent, the father had said that he was unhappy with the service, unhappy with Crista, and did not want Poppy to continue being seen: were the parents allowed to have this child discharged? Monica side-stepped the personal complaint against her colleague, but said truthfully but unwittingly that it was the parent's decision to have their child discharged just as it was within their gift to give consent, with the added rider that they should absolutely discuss this with the therapist and the school, as although the parents may not be able to see the progress their child was making, the school and the therapist may be able to demonstrate it.

It was now clear that the father in the scenario was potentially manipulating both Crista and Monica, and trying to avoid close scrutiny from and contact with the professionals involved. Once this question had been raised, Monica knew she should have set up a meeting with Crista immediately following that first session to discuss how to manage the boundaries of this case. Although their paths rarely crossed, efforts should have been made, by email or phone if face-to-face contact was not possible. Part of her anger was anger at herself for breaching her own professional code when she should have known better.

On the surface, each practitioner had 'merely' offered general information to the parents and avoided discussing a child who was neither their patient nor known to them in any way. However, the ramifications included undermining months of hard work on both sides, with potentially major child protection issues.

Crista and Monica did get together to discuss the incident and future management. As part of the discussion, the following issues arose.

➤ The need for absolute case confidentiality, and for each child to be considered in isolation.

➤ The need for an assertive response: 'Unfortunately I can only discuss the child I am responsible for. Please do contact your own therapist if you have any questions about X.'

➤ The need to make notes about 'coffee' discussions as these may be required as time-line evidence in future safeguarding discussions.

➤ The need to note as a clinical incident, to discuss with the line manager, and to decide how to pre-empt future difficulties: by having a case conference? By not sharing the caseload? How to manage this practically.

Patients are located in a complex web: it maybe helpful to draw a web showing who is part of it and who we need to consider here.

> **Scenario 3**[15]
> A Sure Start programme was considering employing Sam, the parent of a child attending the programme, to do some care work in the venue that her child

---

15 Adapted from *Boundaries*. Available at: www.counsellingconnection.com (accessed April 2013).

attended. In this instance, the employer was considering whether to ignore her instinct to avoid setting up a 'dual relationship', where the employee would also be a beneficiary of the programme.[16]

Considerations Scenario 3

➤ Are dual relationships ever acceptable?
➤ Would it make a difference if Sam was employed at another Sure Start venue in a different part of town?
➤ How would Sam's employment play on the concepts of beneficence (providing benefits) and non-maleficence (avoiding causing harm)?
➤ Is the blurring of boundaries ever beneficial?
➤ What other scenarios can you envisage? What if Sam's own child needed urgent attention while she was case working with another child? How would other parents feel about her being employed?
➤ Consider the ramifications if a GP practice employed a patient as a member of staff.

Discussion Scenario 3

Employing Sam could honour her autonomy, self-determination, and her worth and dignity, while also helping to support the family economically, although it is debatable whether this is the role of a Sure Start programme. On the other hand, the values of privacy, the well-being of the child and parents, human relationships, integrity, service, and equality could potentially be contravened. The decision to employ also potentially diminishes beneficence, non-maleficence and utilitarianism (an action is right if it produces the greatest good for the greatest number) since the blurring of boundaries may not be in the best interests of the other parents in the programme. We need to consider which 'actions are right or wrong according to the balance of their good and bad consequences'.[17]

For this, we need to apply proportion, weighing up the benefits of each. Potential good could come from the employment, outweighing the potential bad effect, possibly making it the better of the two options. There is a recognition that the choice to employ is not always going to result in positive outcomes, but allows that it is better to decide on the option that produces the least harm: the autonomy, worth and dignity of the person are enhanced by allowing the parent to choose on her or his own behalf. This option also maximises the well-being of the children, the general well-being of the parent, the well-being of the employer and the well-being of the staff. The employer's integrity is maintained

---

16 Bader E. Dual relationships: legal and ethical trends. *Transactional Analysis*. 1994; **24**(1): 64–6. Reamer FG. Boundary issues in social work: managing dual relationships. *Social Work*. 2003; **48**: 121–32.
17 Beauchamp, Childress, note 9 above, p. 47.

while providing quality services and acting in a trustworthy manner. The employer is endeavouring to act for the benefit of others and to do no harm.

However, if the correct boundaries, listed below, are put in place, the decision to employ Sam is suddenly easy, possible, ethical and boundaried.

➤ If Sam was employed under strict equal opportunities legislation, that is, if the appointment was open to the public and any of the parents in the programme were able to apply

➤ If she was employed after an organisational consultation and policy approval process.

➤ If the employer met with her regularly to support her role as a parent while also helping her to develop her professional skills.

➤ If she was encouraged to remain actively involved in the programme that her child attended.

➤ If she was supported in dealing with issues of role conflict that arose, such as what to do when her daughter was ill and had to remain home when Sam was due at work.

➤ If all parties were clear about the different relationships: Sam's with her case manager, with her co-workers, with the other parents enrolled in her child's programme, and other parents involved in the programme overall.

➤ If general guidelines and policies were established to ensure that the ensuing dual relationships were neither exploitive nor harmful.

By far the best option to support the employer, employee and other clients would be to develop specific employment hiring and interview policies, not simply one that supported or banned dual relationships. These would support the ethical conduct of the employer and protect it should problems arise. For example, one guideline could be that parents would not be employed to work in the same setting as their child, or that the programme would only employ parents from a local, non-affiliated Sure Start and that the programme would refer parents interested in employment opportunities to this separate one. This clear boundary would mean that:

➤ parents could still be accepted for employment without establishing dual relationships as illustrated above

➤ all parents would be free to apply for the available positions

➤ employment law is followed

➤ the quality of the services is maintained by the right of the employer not to hire the parent if he or she is not determined to be a good fit

➤ parents who were unable to navigate the confidentiality issues raised by dual relationships would not be hired.

Of course, the very best option is that the parent would not be working in the same setting as her or his child, as then issues of equality are addressed, the well-being of the enrolled children is ensured and role conflict issues are diminished. Sam would be freer to meet the needs of the children in her care, without wanting to give more attention to her own child. However, the well-being of the parents is also supported by recognising that employment in the programme may be beneficial for some parents but not for others. The overall integrity and trustworthiness of the employer is maintained because it is acceptable for it to utilise its free choice in deciding to begin or to not begin a dual relationship. If procedures are followed, this would be a possible option, but may be a risky one. It would be crucial to build a body of policies and guidelines for the employer to follow in the future as the major limitation of this option is that the potential for inequality exists. If parents are not treated equally, the definition of standards over time could prove to be unethical.

Ultimately, clinical pragmatism and reflective practice dictates, but we do need to consider what is best for a particular individual *and* what is best for the group. Ethical decision making involves continuous reflection and self-awareness.[18] It would be thoughtful and helpful to employ Sam, but a more pragmatic, possibly assertive, stance revolves around the use of consensus.[19] In this option, which is safer, consensus could be incorporated into the hiring decision process by involving the employer's line manager, so the employer receives the guidance in coming to a determination, rather than making a unilateral decision.

Anyone with an ongoing clinical caseload has to assert boundaries and model how to observe the rules. We are much more aware now of the need to develop appropriate boundaries in our clinical work with patients. For example, doctors are aware of the need to protect their professional integrity by having chaperones available during personal medical examinations. Psychotherapists and counsellors have developed a clear therapeutic framework,[20] which includes not touching, as it may be misconstrued, and other lines of behaviour that must not be crossed – by the therapist or the client, or both. In this context, the theory of boundaries has grown up around work with survivors of sexual abuse. While it is helpful and clarifying in that context, it has since been developed to extend to thinking around issues such as fees (which must be set out in advance), telephone/texting contact between sessions (not advised as it can encourage over-dependency) and the importance of keeping to agreed session times. By asserting these boundaries both the patient/client and the practitioner are protected.

---

18 Mattison M. Ethical decision making: the person in the process. *Social Work*. 2000; **45**: 201–12.
19 Fins JJ, Bacchetta MD, Miller FG. Clinical pragmatism: a method of moral problem solving. *Kennedy Institute of Ethics Journal*. 1997; **7**(2): 129–43.
20 Totton, note 2 above.

Many therapists have written about the ground rules which are fundamental to those working independently in private practice;[21] these apply equally to any practitioner working within or independently of the NHS. Indeed, many of the rules have now been subsumed into our contracts of employment in the NHS. A variety of different professional bodies have their own rules (e.g. Canadian Counselling Association, 2007; Association for Addiction Professionals NAADAC, 2008), but they are very similar. Again, these ideally need to be in the form of a written agreement which includes the following.

Formal structures
➤ Determining role clarification and seeking informed consent through consultation and documentation.
➤ Appointments having a set time and place.
➤ If payments are involved, having a set, non-negotiable fee and payment terms defined: never barter fees as this will blur boundaries.
➤ No giving and receiving of gifts; if gifts are given, the act needs to be recorded.
➤ Confidentiality within the session, only broken under agreed terms that protect the client or anyone else from risk of harm.

Understood structures
➤ To have an entirely professional, not emotional or sexual, involvement with patients/clients.
➤ No telephone contact with patients between sessions unless strictly necessary and pre-arranged.
➤ No social relationships with clients, including internet contact, for example, on Facebook.
➤ Avoiding duel/multiple roles, for example, being both the client's employer and their professional support.
➤ To prevent potential abuse and harm, and to protect patients and clients from exploitation: remember, you are in a position of power, and the patients are vulnerable in this situation.
➤ To avoid any conflict of interest, in whatever form.

These important boundaries help to make patients feel safe, held; it helps their trust. The minute these are abused or allowed to vary, problems can set in: what

---

21 Smith DL. *Hidden Conversations: introduction to communicative psychoanalysis.* Routledge; 1991. Zur O. To cross or not to cross: do boundaries in therapy protect or harm? *Psychotherapy Bulletin.* 2004; **39**(3): 27–32. Epstein RS, Simon RI. The exploitation index: an early warning indicator of boundary violations in psychotherapy. *Bulletin of the Menniger Clinic.* 1990; **54**: 450–65.

has been termed the 'slippery slope' theory,[22] where boundaries are continually crossed, relaxed or unclear the relationship will deteriorate until it becomes unstable.

> **Scenario 4**
>
> A parent was allowed to change the normal, clinic appointment format for her teenager to another day and time, outside of normal working hours. Neither parent nor child attended, saying the appointment needed to be in a non-NHS setting. Once permitted to vary the agreement, the parent pushed further, asking for a difficult to reach community setting, which the managers agreed. Again, neither attended, so the two attending clinicians had a doubly expensive visit – both by now had cancelled clinics, both spent a morning travelling unnecessarily, both suspecting, rightly, that the appointment would not be attended. The parent nevertheless complained that the service had been unresponsive to her needs and had not provided the care sought for her.

Considerations Scenario 4

➤ How would you have handled this situation?
➤ Would it make a difference if the patient was a younger child?
➤ Who would you approach for guidance if you disagreed with your line manager's decision making here?
➤ Is the blurring of such boundaries ever beneficial, and, if so, how?

Discussion Scenario 4

Two line managers were involved in taking a decision in this scenario. The first advised not to make an appointment outside the NHS setting available, the other felt as the service was a community service they should be seen to be flexible and offer care anywhere in the community: other patients were seen in local community settings such as children's centres, schools and GP practices.

However, the two clinicians involved felt that once a boundary had been breached, the patient was bound to push for more. Here, the parent may appear manipulative, but this is unwitting, at least unconscious, for the parent is un-boundaried, and would benefit from another adult – the person in charge – to hold the line. The clinicians involved felt it was therefore crucial for the professional in charge to be seen to set and hold a boundary, so that they could both represent and model how to do so, and demonstrate how things work better when this is done. If the professional is unable to hold the line, the patient may feel lost, formless, unsafe. The boundaries collapsed when pushed, and the two clinicians felt this should not have been permitted.

---

22 Zur, note 21 above. Epstein, Simon, note 21 above.

Assertiveness and adhering to our professional responsibilities[23]

Professionally, we have a responsibility to ourselves, our clients and our colleagues to adhere to certain principles to allow for mutual trust and respect. Behaving assertively, honestly, clearly, ethically and morally can help us uphold those values.

We have a responsibility to work within our own limitations

Professionally, we need to be responsible and assertive about looking after ourselves so that we satisfy the responsibility to provide a competently delivered service that meets the client's needs.

➤ As practitioners, we need to ensure that we are appropriately supported and accountable. To this end, we need to give careful consideration to the limitations of our training and experience and work within these limits, taking advantage of available professional support. If our work with people requires the provision of supervision, we must ensure that we make every effort to attend, as we have no professional defence if we do not push for what we need nor attend what is offered.

➤ We must be assertive about saying 'no' when we feel we have reached the limits of our ability. If we feel unqualified to provide a level of service, or feel unwell or unable to practise safely, for whatever reason, we must be clear about this and withdraw from working, and seek appropriate professional support and services as the need arises. Attending to one's own well-being is essential to sustaining good practice.

➤ We have a responsibility to ourselves to ensure that our work does not become detrimental to our health or well-being by making sure that the way that we undertake our work is as safe as possible.

➤ To maintain competent practice, we should regularly review our need for professional and personal support and obtain appropriate services for ourselves. This is our responsibility, not that of our employers. Regularly monitoring and reviewing one's work is essential to maintaining good practice. It is important to be open to, and conscientious in considering, feedback from colleagues, appraisals, training and assessments. Responding constructively to feedback helps to advance practice. Committing to good practice requires us to keep up to date with the latest knowledge and respond to changing circumstances.

➤ Assertive practice involves clarifying and agreeing the rights and responsibilities of both the practitioner and the client at appropriate points in their working relationship, not fudging issues or passively being led by another's agenda.

➤ We must be proactive, and ensure that records are accurate, do not include

---

23 Expanded and abridged from www.bacp.co.uk (accessed May 2013).

irrelevant or personal opinion, are respectful of clients and colleagues, and are protected from unauthorised disclosure.

➤ We must be clear about any legal requirements concerning our work, and consider them conscientiously and be legally accountable for their practice.

We have a responsibility to gain and honour the trust of clients

Keeping trust requires that we are always open and honest in our dealings with all people, and that we remain clear about our working principles. Thus patients/clients need to know, and be reassured, of the following.

➤ Their needs may be reviewed by the practitioner and others. These reviews may be conducted, when appropriate, in consultation with clients, supervisors, managers or other practitioners with relevant expertise.

➤ Practitioners will remain attentive to the quality of listening and respect offered to them, and ensure culturally appropriate ways of communicating that are courteous and clear and demonstrate respect for privacy and dignity

➤ Practitioners will respect their right to choose whether to continue or withdraw.

➤ Practitioners understand issues of capacity and consent: that working with young people requires specific ethical awareness and competence. Here, practitioners are required to consider and assess the balance between the young person's dependence on adults and carers and their progressive development towards acting independently. Working with children and young people requires careful consideration of issues concerning their capacity to give consent to receiving any service independently of someone with parental responsibilities and the management of confidences disclosed by clients.

➤ Practitioners have a professional duty to respond to clients' requests for information about the way they are working and any assessment that they may have made. This professional requirement does not apply if it is considered that imparting this information would be detrimental to the client or inconsistent with the approach previously agreed with the client. Clients may have legal rights to this information, and these need to be taken into account.

➤ Practitioners do not abuse their client's trust in order to gain sexual, emotional, financial or any other kind of personal advantage. Practitioners should think carefully about, and exercise considerable caution before, entering into personal or business relationships with former clients and should expect to be professionally accountable if the relationship becomes detrimental to the client or the standing of the profession.

➤ Practitioners do not allow their professional relationships with clients to be prejudiced by any personal views they may hold about lifestyle, gender, age, disability, race, sexual orientation, beliefs or culture.

➤ Practitioners should be clear about any commitment to be available to clients and colleagues and honour these commitments.

➤ Conflicts of interest are best avoided, provided they can be reasonably foreseen in the first instance and prevented from arising. In deciding how to respond to conflicts of interest, the protection of the client's interests and maintaining their trust in the practitioner should be paramount.

We have a responsibility to protect our clients from forseeable harm

Practitioners must behave quickly and assertively if they have good reason to believe that a colleague is placing a patient at risk of harm. They have a responsibility to raise any concerns with the practitioner concerned in the first instance, unless it is inappropriate to do so. If the matter cannot be resolved, they should review the grounds for their concern and the evidence available to them and, when appropriate, raise their concerns with the practitioner's manager, agency or professional body. If a practitioner is uncertain what to do, their concerns should be discussed with an experienced colleague or a supervisor, or raised with their professional association, which will be able to advice on professional conduct procedures.

We have a responsibility to work in harmony with our colleagues

Professional relationships should be conducted in a spirit of mutual respect. Practitioners should try to maintain good working relationships and systems of communication that enhance services to clients at all times. For this, we need to be aware of some ground rules.

➤ Practitioners should treat all colleagues fairly and foster equality opportunity.

➤ Practitioners should not allow their professional relationships with colleagues to be prejudiced by their own personal views about a colleague's lifestyle, gender, age, disability, race, sexual orientation, beliefs or culture. It is unacceptable and unethical to discriminate against colleagues on any of these grounds.

➤ Practitioners must not undermine a colleague's relationships with clients by making unjustified or unsustainable comments.

➤ All communications between colleagues about clients should be on a professional basis and thus purposeful, respectful and consistent with the management of confidences as declared to clients.

Personal moral qualities

The practitioner's personal moral qualities are of crucial importance to those we work with. Many of the personal qualities considered important in the provision of services have an ethical or moral component and are therefore considered as virtues, or good personal qualities. We cannot demand that all practitioners possess these qualities, since this is impracticable: it is better that the qualities are deeply rooted in the person concerned and developed out of personal commitment rather than the requirement of an external authority. Personal qualities to which caring or healthcare professionals are strongly encouraged to aspire include some of those excellent communication skills we discussed in the first section of this book. Through maturity, learning and personal development, we may develop some of these skills.[24]

- ➤ **Empathy:** the ability to communicate understanding of another person's experience from that person's perspective.
- ➤ **Sincerity:** a personal commitment to consistency between what is professed and what is done.
- ➤ **Integrity:** commitment to being moral in dealings with others, personal straightforwardness, honesty and coherence.
- ➤ **Resilience:** the capacity to work with the client's concerns without being personally diminished.
- ➤ **Respect:** showing appropriate esteem to others and their understanding of themselves.
- ➤ **Humility:** the ability to assess accurately and acknowledge one's own strengths and weaknesses.
- ➤ **Competence:** the effective deployment of the skills and knowledge needed to do what is required.
- ➤ **Fairness:** the consistent application of appropriate criteria to inform decisions and actions.
- ➤ **Wisdom:** the possession of sound judgement that informs practice.
- ➤ **Courage:** the capacity to act in spite of known fears, risks and uncertainty.

To work ethically is very challenging, and requires constant self-reflection and analysis. As we saw in the scenarios above, we will inevitably encounter situations where there are competing obligations. At such times, it might be tempting to retreat from analysis in order to escape a sense of what may appear to be unresolvable ethical tension. But this would be cowardly and passive. There are always alternative points of view and, providing we can justify our clinical reasoning, it is understood that we are making professional judgements in good faith, in circumstances that may be constantly changing and full of uncertainties. We need to be able to demonstrate that we understand, and are committing ourselves to engaging with, the challenge of striving to be ethical, even when doing so involves making difficult decisions. It is then we are seen to be acting courageously.

---

24 *See* note 23 above.

KEY POINTS

➤ In ethical dilemmas, there are always good and bad consequences, never clear-cut solutions, but healthy compromises need to be reached. There will be a wrong way, a right way and another way. Nothing is prescriptive.

➤ Each perspective is motivated by personal, professional and organisational interests. Withdraw from the situation and move from your own partial view to gain an overall view.

➤ As clinicians, we follow some fundamental ground rules when we work, which help keep the patient, and us, safe. In developing ground rules, a boundary, we tell our patients: 'This is yours, and this is mine'; we tell them what they, and we, are responsible for.

➤ The purpose of having boundaries as a clinician is to protect and take care of ourselves, in order to give the best service we can without being contaminated with our own issues, and also to set the limits that help to support others to trust us.

➤ We also need to consider the demands of practice, legislation, registration and the recognition of our competencies. This is the core stuff of risk management: if we can demonstrate that we self-monitor, reflect, question, consider and, where necessary, seek support for our decision making (through accurate note keeping, supervision records, etc.) we are much better placed.

➤ We need to find ways of working that are based on giving the patient the best therapy, best suited to them, rather than being forced to work defensively, in ways to avoid vulnerability to criticism or disciplinary hearings.

➤ Respect the safeguarding agenda and the patient's right to be self-determining and enable them to make their own decisions. Consider who has the authority for making the decision: always consider and re-consider your own autonomy, authority and accountability for making and acting on decisions.

➤ Boundaries are guidelines that are founded on the basic principles of clinical codes of ethics. These include informed consent, open discussion, consultation, supervision, documentation, actions which produce the greatest good for the greatest number and examination of personal motivation.

➤ Boundaries are a crucial aspect of any effective clinician/client/patient relationship. They set the structure for the relationship and provide a consistent framework for the treatment process. What we are aiming for is something suited to the patient/clients' changing needs and circumstances, not rigid, inflexible boundaries/guidelines, nor too much flexibility so both parties become enmeshed and neither understands the boundary.

➤ If challenged by a situation, consider the challenges of confidentiality, responsibilities, professionalism, privacy, loyalties and consent. If unsure, discuss with colleagues. In the light of your discussion, are the decisions you make effective, efficient and equitable? Think about whose emotions are evoked, whose need is being met. Are your responses emotional or professional, and does it matter?

➤ To keep our practice safe we need to:
  – work within our own limitations
  – gain the trust of clients
  – work in harmony with our colleagues
  – uphold personal, moral qualities of empathy, sincerity, integrity, resilience, respect, humility, competence, fairness, wisdom and courage: the capacity to act in spite of known fears, risks and uncertainty.

FURTHER READING

Bond T. *Standards and Ethics for Counselling in Action*. 3rd ed. Counselling in Action series. Sage; 2009.

Corey G, Corey MS, Callanan P. *Issues and Ethics in the Helping Professions*. Brooks/Cole Publishing Co.; 1998.

Fry S, Johnstone MJ. *Ethics in Nursing Practice: a guide to ethical decision making*. 3rd ed. Wiley-Blackwell; 2008.

Hawley G. *Ethics in Clinical Practice: an inter-professional approach*. Pearson Education; 2007.

Howatson-Jones L. *Reflective Practice in Nursing*. Transforming Nursing Practice series. Learning Matters; 2010.

Jackson J. *Ethics in Medicine*. Polity Press; 2000.

Jackson J. *Truth, Trust and Medicine*. Routledge; 2001.

National Association of Social Workers (United States). *Code of Ethics of the National Association of Social Workers*. National Association of Social Workers; 1999. Available at: www.socialworker.com (accessed April 2013).

Parrot L. *Values and Ethics in Social Work Practice*. Transforming Social Work Practice series. Learning Matters; 2006.

Pope KS, Vasquez MJ. *Ethics in Psychotherapy and Counseling: a practical guide for psychologists*. Jossey-Bass Publishers; 1991.

Reamer FG. *Social Work Values and Ethics*. Columbia University Press; 1995.

Section 4

Applying assertiveness skills

CHAPTER 15

Your personal development plan

Personal development improves self-awareness and self-knowledge. It can help to build or renew personal identity, develop strengths and talents, and identify or improve potential. Through reading this book, and taking the exercises seriously, you will be improving your personal autonomy and social skills. Personal development is also about establishing identity; developing competence, purpose, integrity and mature interpersonal relationships; managing emotions; and achieving autonomy and interdependence.[1]

This final section explores some of the ways it is possible to continue with self-development and fulfil aspirations, through being assertive, setting goals and managing change.

The concept of personal development covers a wider field than self-development or self-help: personal development also includes developing other people. This may take place through roles such as those of a teacher or mentor, manager or clinician. In my sister volume, *Developing Leadership Skills for Health and Social Care Professionals*, we explore using personal development plans as part of developing management and leadership skills, but here we look at some of the competencies required to apply assertiveness skills to develop yourself and your relationships at home and at work – with family, friends, patients, clients and colleagues.

If you know yourself better, you are more likely to be able to take control of your life, and to live it actively rather than passively. As you behave more assertively, a different kind of respect is demanded and earned. Those unused to this new role may need to learn new personal skills to support their new sense of self.

EXERCISE 1

➤ Does your life provide you with opportunities for growth and learning?
➤ What are you plans for the next five, or 15, years?

---

1 Chickering A, Reisser L. *Education and Identity*. Jossey-Bass; 1993.

➤ How much personal authority do you have?

➤ Do you feel that you are making a worthwhile contribution?

KEY SKILLS

To continue to develop, you need to practise your newly learnt skills, and be open to, and take the time to, talk with people so that vital relationships can grow. Learn from these connections; look at what others around you are doing and locate the key qualities and skills that you most respect and value. What are the qualities in these people? Diplomacy? Enthusiasm? Confidence? Compassion? Ability to motivate? Kindness? Competence? Clarity? If you question friends and colleagues about valued personal qualities, they will often cite kindness, humour, respect, good listening skills, empathy, foresight, flexibility, generosity and tolerance. Good team workers and practitioners also demonstrate good problem-solving, decision-making and assertiveness skills.

Have you got these skills? Do you want to change? If so, look at some of these skills and develop them.

➤ Personal development refers to the methods and systems that support self-development and may include: improving self-awareness, self-knowledge, personal, spiritual and professional strengths, talents, and potential.

➤ Personal development can include developing yourself and others through teaching, mentoring, counselling, therapy, couching, supervising.

➤ Team working requires good problem-solving ability, and a capacity to tolerate each other's working styles. In this situation, you both keep checking your tolerances and expectations of each other. The skills required are those of collaboration and a sense of healthy, managed competition.

➤ In developing our own people skills, we need to network, listen and plan ahead. For this we need knowledge, motivation, tolerance and behavioural skills such as assertiveness, communication, influencing skills, complex cognitive abilities, self-knowledge, emotional resilience and personal drive.

Experience suggests that it is good to develop *problem-solving* skills alongside assertiveness skills, where you devise a technique to arrive at solutions. If the problem involves a direct work situation, make a decision based on your experience; if not, use other people's experience to assist: discuss problems and their solutions collectively. Your forte is to be able to recognise the solution and 'decide' on it; you do not have to have the answers, just the ability to find them. Be assertive and act: never ignore problems, but take appropriate steps. If *mistakes* are made, point them out but allow for an explanation. Accept certain mistakes as inevitable; look for a solution together. Be *flexible*, maintain a sense of the outside world and understand that the world, and people, is not always perfect.

If in work you have to make *uncomfortable decisions*, do not allow guilt to invade the issue. It only places you in a vulnerable position and you may make concessions you will come to regret. Do not moralise or try to justify your actions, but keep accurate documentation of the incidents that led you to your decision. Stop being *timid*. Either trust your own judgement or tackle your fear of being disliked. There is no place in our busy workplaces for a worker who cannot say 'no'.

Be assertive

➤ Do not avoid difficult situations or accept mediocrity.
➤ Face your insecurities, and learn how to cope with authority.
➤ Listen, ask questions, take advice and then *act*.
➤ Allow yourself to make mistakes – assurance will come with experience.
➤ Remember that there is no such thing as perfection.
➤ Bring yourself into the best focus possible.
➤ Remember that good intentions are as important as any other quality.
➤ Take the responsibility and use all your capabilities.

PLAN YOUR LIFE

In this section, we consider how to plan ahead effectively. These skills can be used by yourself in life planning, and also by patients and clients as they come to make changes in their own lives.

It is said that in life there are four types of people:
➤ people who watch things happen
➤ people to whom things happen
➤ people who do not know what is happening
➤ people who make things happen.

If you are concerned for your future, or feel you are limiting yourself, give yourself some time to reflect and answer the following questions.

EXERCISE 2

Who: mentally scan all the people who may be helpful to you in reaching your personal goals.
What: are the key areas you can tackle quickly?
Where: reflect on your current work and living environment.
When: timing is crucial. When to act or not is a highly developed skill.
How: think about new, creative and innovative actions. Trust your intuition. The behaviour that caused the problem is unlikely to solve it.
Why: think about your own needs.

➤ Do you pay sufficient attention to your personal needs?

➤ What support is available and do you use it well?

➤ What pressures do you inflict on yourself and your family?

➤ Who controls how you use your time?

➤ What recent changes are affecting you most and how?

➤ In which areas of life do you feel most comfortable and uncomfortable?

➤ What are your expectations and constraints?

➤ How have you changed over the past year?

➤ What did you achieve?

➤ What would you like to do more of?

EXERCISE 3

From answering these questions, what changes do you need to make?

1

2

3

4

5

Look back to Section 1, Chapter 3 for some of the ideas, influences and motivating factors to consider when planning ahead for yourself.

EXERCISE 4[2]

Consider and review the following areas of your life. How satisfied are you currently with this area of your life? Give yourself a mark out of 10. For each, write down your lifetime goal, short-term goal (the year ahead), what you want in terms of outcome, and consider the losses and gains in achieving that goal. What are you doing towards meeting that goal? Think about the following considerations.

➤ The goals must be SMART, and stated positively.

➤ Is it within your control to do this?

➤ Describe the context.

- Who else will be involved?
- Why are you doing it?
- What, specifically, do you want the outcome to be?
- Where will you do it? When? How?

---

2 Ready R, Burton K. *Neurolinguistic Programming for Dummies.* John Wiley & Sons; 2004. Ch. 3, p. 43.

➤ Have you identified any resources needed?
➤ Is it ecologically smart?
➤ Have you identified the first step to take?
➤ How will you know the outcome? Evoke your senses: will you be able to see/smell/taste/touch/hear or feel it?
➤ Identify secondary gains.
  – What is the real purpose of this?
  – Whose need am I meeting?
  – What will I lose or gain if I reach my goal?
  – What will happen if I achieve it or not?
  – What will not happen if I do not achieve it?
➤ What will the reward be?
  – Focus on the benefits of success.
➤ Tell friends what you are doing, so they can help and assist.
➤ Keep a diary of progress and revisit monthly.

Areas of life to consider

		Date	Lifetime	Short term	Outcome	Gains	Losses	What doing?
Home environment	/10							
Money	/10							
Spiritual values	/10							
Emotional health	/10							
Creativity	/10							
The environment	/10							
Work	/10							
Friendships	/10							
Family	/10							
Health	/10							
Recreation/leisure	/10							
Other								

MANAGING YOUR RELATIONSHIPS ASSERTIVELY

You have to decide when it is possible, and practical, to ask people for help and when to turn elsewhere, then you will not be victimised by the real, or imagined, failings of others. If you feel people – friends, family, colleagues – no longer listen or communicate well and are no longer *accessible*, you may feel overlooked and ignored. Consider that you may have disappointed or dissatisfied them and they have unassertively begun withdrawing their attention. Here they are not being assertive, so you have to take the lead and solicit constructive criticism: ask; identify the problem. Be assertive and offer solutions; exercise your own initiative. It will strengthen your relationships.

Learn to qualify and quantify your own, and your family's, life and productivity. Assess yourself as a unit and so increase your efficiency and effectiveness. Meet informally to confront difficult situations and solve problems, together. Make it an annual review, where you review your lives together, using the above chart. Use the time to check that you understand each other and are happy with these areas of your life, together and alone. Listen well, confront difficult situations and solve problems, together.

If you are afraid to admit to mistakes, remember that errors are inevitable. Women especially have a problem believing this, and hesitate to jump in without preparation, afraid of making a mistake. Men, however, are socialised to be more confident, so go through a time of error-making to acquire their expertise. From an early age, women's efforts are more focused on avoiding the errors that bring criticism. If this is the case, begin by acquiring as much experience as you can, and, if you make an error, devise strategies to cover yourself. Learning from your errors is an important way of acquiring wisdom. Act quickly: do not procrastinate, as mistakes are better tolerated when people see that you understand your error and that you have taken steps to correct it. If you have made the mistake of not dealing with a problem immediately, act as if the delay had never occurred.

Take charge and plan your life so that it fulfils *your* capacities, needs and dreams, not those of other people. For this you need to be able to discriminate, be analytical and be honest with yourself.

➤ What are your dreams? Where do you want to see yourself?
➤ What are your strengths, your assets?
➤ What are your weaknesses? What areas do you need to strengthen yourself in? What areas of knowledge or self-cultivation must you pursue?
➤ What kind of lifestyle do you wish to achieve?

To achieve your goals, you will need knowledge, assertiveness, communication and influencing skills, motivation, self-knowledge, emotional resilience and personal drive. Cultivate them if you wish to succeed, and apply your newly found knowledge and skills to develop your relationships with everyone you meet.

KEY POINTS

➤ Personal development improves self-awareness and self-knowledge. It can help to build or renew personal identity, develop strengths and talents, identify or improve potential, and fulfil aspirations. It can help to improve your relationships at home and work, with family, friends, patients, clients and colleagues.
➤ Personal development refers to the methods and systems that support self-development, and may include improving self awareness, self-knowledge, personal, spiritual and professional strengths, talents and potential.

➤ If you know yourself better, you are more likely to be able to take control of your life, and live it actively rather than passively. As you behave more assertively, a different kind of respect is demanded and earned.

➤ In order to develop, one skill is to review your life, and check that it provides you with the necessary opportunities for growth and learning, over the long and short term.

➤ Learn the key skills from your connections. Look at the valued personal qualities in those you love and learn from them. Use this knowledge to change yourself.

➤ Experience suggests that it is good to develop problem-solving skills, accepting and learning from mistakes, being flexible, maintaining a sense of the outside world, and understanding that the world, and people, are not always perfect.

➤ Plan your life: make things happen. Consider your lifetime and short-term goals, what you want in terms of outcome, the losses and gains in achieving those goals. What are you doing towards meeting each goal? Identify the secondary gains and the rewards, and revisit regularly.

➤ Manage your relationships assertively. Do not be afraid of asking for help. Take the lead and solicit constructive criticism. Ask; identify the problem. Share problem solving.

➤ Take charge and plan your life so it fulfills *your* capacities, needs and dreams, not those of other people. Be honest with yourself. Look critically at your strengths and weaknesses. What areas do you need to strengthen yourself in? What areas of knowledge or self-cultivation must you pursue? To achieve your goals, you will need assertiveness skills, motivation self-knowledge, emotional resilience and personal drive.

FURTHER READING

Ready R, Burton K. *Neurolinguistic Programming for Dummies*. John Wiley & Sons; 2004.

CHAPTER 16

Goal setting and supporting change

You will by now have a clear idea about what assertiveness is and how to be assertive. You will have practiced some of the key skills and faced some challenges. You will, in some areas of your life, be putting some of those skills into practice. In this final chapter we look at how to accept and manage change, to plan ahead and set goals: the skills that can be both used by you and taught to clients.

You will be changed by the process of learning to be assertive. These changes may challenge you, or your clients, families and friends. The goals may be small, as in using newly learnt assertiveness skills to say 'no' to a colleague, or bigger, such as challenging a superior at work. In Chapter 4 we looked at setting goals and managing change; here we look in more detail at what those changes may mean and what the obstacles to change are.

Modern life requires us to adapt, and learn fast. Life, relationships and work all change in both style and content. We all thus need to be proactive rather than reactive, so that change is anticipated and planned. To make change successful for ourselves and our clients, we need to develop an awareness of what makes change possible, the barriers to change and what is needed to make changes, especially in ourselves and our behaviours.

There is no magic formula for change management, but there are some clear themes, which include having a clear sense of direction and the ability to be experimental, creative, flexible and prepared to take risks.

Our patients and clients too need to work hard to understand the need for change, to take on board the need to manage all or part of their own care and, as we saw in Section 3, the need to take responsibility for managing themselves and their condition. This chapter explores the personal and professional skills needed to manage the process of change, for yourself and for your clients. Here we focus on the professional challenges; the managerial and leadership challenges are explored in my sister volume, *Developing Leadership Skills for Health and Social Care Professionals*.

MANAGING CHANGE

Change is an inescapable part of our lives, and yet most people resist change. Consider the following.

➤ What is change?
➤ Why do we need to change?
➤ How can we overcome resistance to change?
➤ How can we manage change and set goals?

Change is a constant in the workplace and world – to survive, and grow, we must adjust to change. Change is also messy, and risky. Just when you think you have arrived, you find that you have hardly begun. Change is the key to progress, but we resist it, because people react differently to change and change can be unsettling. It pays to be proactive, since if we assume no change, or try to escape it, our choices will be harsher. We need to adapt to a turbulent world. We need to be less passive and embrace change, and take part in setting the goals: then we are empowered to alter our own futures. This is where assertiveness comes in.

Change has to be managed and, as with any process, it needs to be understood before it can be managed. We need to prepare for:

➤ how to plan for change
➤ how to implement change
➤ how to evaluate change.

Within this, we need to identify both the future that we desire and some of the forces driving change, plus our own reactions to change and the size and shape of the work to be done.

Step 1: Understanding the need for change

Change is both fundamental to progress and necessary for survival. We need to understand and present the positive reasons for change, to counter the resistance.

Step 2: Understanding resistance

Change is always problematic because it presents dilemmas and conflict between:

➤ the need to experiment versus the need to be right
➤ managing the present versus managing the change
➤ managing uncertainty versus certainty
➤ the ease of status quo versus innovation.

In personal change, which we are addressing here, there are changes to both external and internal lives as skills are learnt and lives re-shared. This can be threatening to people. There are no simple answers. Balances need to be struck, without compromising principles. We need to understand that resistance to change is often the expression of insecurity and fear: it exposes people to uncertainty and may alter relationships and patterns of behaviour for the worse. It is therefore more acceptable when the objectives and application are understood and do not offer a threat to security.

What individual resistance to change do we know about?

EXERCISE 1

What are your own reasons not to change?

No time	Previously tried, it did not work	It's not in the plan
Habit	Inconvenience	Own (biased) view of situation
Loss of individualisation	Cost of change	Threat to self
Financial implication	Everyone will blame me if it doesn't work	
Fear of being disliked	Fear of the unknown	Loss of security

Look at these and see which character you are,[1] and see whether you can identify your patient/client. If you can see a pattern, use the chosen techniques to persuade and support the change.

EXERCISE 2

➤ Hares: progressive, adventurous, believe in professionalism and best practice. In discussing change, emphasise logic and evidence.
➤ Dinosaurs: reactionary, dissatisfied, resistant to change, old-fashioned. To support through change, show deference and respect, give support and sympathy.
➤ Sheep: conservative, traditional, conscientious, caring, avoid risk. In supporting, show respect, emphasise that this behaviour is standard, normal practice.
➤ Wolves: entrepreneurs, active, energetic, ambitious. They love change. Wolves do not need support, but encouragement: emphasise any dynamic aspects of change and the benefits to the their health, home and professional life.

---

1 *Practice Manager*. 2000.

How do you, and your clients, react to change? Do you and they feel confident and excited or uncertain and frightened?

Step 3: Identify the need for change
➤ Stay alert to the need for change.
➤ Consider where you are now.
➤ Consider where you want to be.

Step 4: Plan ahead for big changes
Effective change needs careful planning. Any personal change will affect those close to you, and they may feel threatened. At this stage you need to identify who will be opposed and therefore not assist; identify who will not oppose but will not assist; and, to gain support, who will want it to happen, and make it happen. Recognise where there is agreement and conflict, and examine your own/your client's further training needs.

EXERCISE 3

If your client is planning a big change, which will have a big impact, and they feel overwhelmed, discuss the implications visually. Chart who you need to involve, highlighting those who will support or challenge the change, by placing those involved as spokes around the hub of a wheel, or a mind map. There are many smart phone 'apps'[2] that you and your client could use to help in the mind-mapping process. Here we look at supporting a client with a house move.

Moving house
The move will enable some, and create problems for others. Note the positives and negatives for each family member.

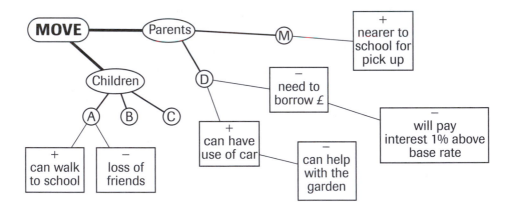

---

2   See iMindMap or SimpleMind+ for examples.

Step 5: Make the change, and make it successful

Experiment. Be dynamic. Change is successful where it has been preceded by other successful changes. Take charge, and demonstrate you have the energy, confidence and commitment to carry it through. Successful change is organic and dynamic, and involves innovation and ice-breaking.

Pointers to assist you in managing the change process:

➤ allow for a period of transition
➤ seek commitment and support
➤ seek out role models and friends who support you
➤ problem solve
➤ break things into steps –: what needs to be done, when, by whom
➤ monitor your progress
➤ share your vision, your fundamental beliefs
➤ be honest with yourself
➤ listen to and understand the negatives
➤ acknowledge the history of organising things in a certain way, so any changes can be put on trial to see whether they work
➤ use your supporters' energy, enthusiasm and lead
➤ preserve as many of the existing benefits as possible
➤ make people aware of the inevitable losses as well as the gains
➤ involve your closest colleagues and friends in identifying the need for change, and planning the new
➤ provide facts to avoid rumour and uncertainty
➤ provide reassurance
➤ communicate – keep an open door and an open mind.

Be aware of the effects of too much stress, and the effects of speedy change:

Shock ⟶ defensive withdrawal ⟶ acknowledgement ⟶ adaptation

Allow for and accommodate these feelings, and respond to them by encouraging those affected to seek additional professional support if necessary.

Change can be both painful and unacceptable to those who are not 'change masters'. Here are some pointers:

➤ do not assume that everyone will understand and accept the need for change
➤ explain openly and clearly what you want to do and why, to decrease any anxieties and instabilities
➤ expect people to be surprised or hurt, or to attack or question your intentions
➤ people will express concerns which conflict with your own, but this does not mean that they cannot understand that what you want to do is the best thing – there are people in every age group who are always going to dislike change, however necessary or desirable it is

➤ base your plans on accurate information and predictions
➤ keep to a timetable for plans and their implementation
➤ allow plenty of time for consultation; ask people for their opinions and take notice of their replies
➤ if you have to deal directly with angry interested parties, take their concerns seriously and negotiate – be assertive and open to their influence.

Step 6: Monitor and evaluate

Check that you have accomplished what you set out to do. Should the change be abandoned or adjusted? During the period of change, keep routine life under control. View change as an opportunity, not a threat. We will only learn to master change when we encourage, welcome and incorporate it into our lives. Those who do not fear change grow, learn and continue to develop.

GOAL SETTING

Setting goals helps to develop individual commitment reduce uncertainty in decision making, and help us to focus direction.[3] As we know, we need the goals to tell us where to go, and the objectives to tell us how to get there.

What stops us from achieving goals? Achieving can only happen with good organisation and planning ahead.

Managing change and preventing failure

You will never regret any positive move you make, however small. What you certainly will regret is not trying. Review the SMART goals.
➤ Specific, precise.
➤ Measurable (cost, quality, quantity, timeliness).
➤ Achievable within the timescale.
➤ Realistic (provide a challenge, stretch the employee).
➤ Jointly established not imposed.
➤ Broken down into objectives.
➤ Planned: indicate priorities (must do, could do), subject to a deadline.
➤ Continually updated.
➤ Checked for success.

If a particular task or goal is important enough, it is usually achieved, irrespective of all the obstacles and difficulties. Develop positive and proactive thinking. Here are some tried and tested methods used by counsellors, trainers

---

3   Kast F, Rosenzweig J. *Organisation and Management: a systems and contingency approach.* 4th revised ed. McGraw-Hill; 1985.

and coaches which may support you in achieving your aim. These methods can be used for both personal change/goal setting and managing professional changes. If you find it hard to set goals, be creative, use these ideas to assist you. Copy each exercise and complete one for any professional issues, one for personal development and one for your work-related issues.

EXERCISE 4

Do any of these speak to you? If so, solve the problem.

?

➤ Lack of goals – write them down.
➤ Confusion in priorities – put first things first.
➤ Unrealistic time estimates – allow more time.
➤ Impatience with detail – take time to get it right.
➤ Manage by crisis – develop the skills of discrimination; distinguish between urgent/important.
➤ Over-commitment – take time out, organise yourself.
➤ Indecision – make decisions with incomplete facts.
➤ Fear of the consequences of a mistake – use mistakes as your learning process.

EXERCISE 5

Goals	Personal strengths	Challenges	Development skills	Achievements

This is a useful template to use with clients who are 'stuck', and finding it hard to achieve their goal. Complete this using the following guidelines.

Goals

Goals are the foundation stones. Make them positive: something they want to gain, not something they want to rid themselves of. Describe a goal, not a problem.

Personal strengths

Concentrate on the strengths, not weaknesses. The client needs to believe they are worthy of what they want to achieve. Listing strengths focuses on what is offered.

Immediate challenges/blocks/problems

Focus on problems that directly affect the client – do not list problems that blame or involve other people. Although their goals may well involve X, no one can think or make goals for other people, only for themselves, so do not set: 'To get X to work less hard, then they can pay more attention to my ideas.' Ask the client to consider the problem from another angle: is there a way they can accommodate those long hours? Fill them with something absorbing and stimulating, so the absence bothers them less. Instead of blaming others, ask them to consider their responsibilities – why, for example, they seem to find themselves attracted to people who treat them badly. Then they see the problem in a way that gives them some control over solving it.

Development skills

This is an area for the client to develop and improve. Listing these is a great way to focus on ways the client can move forward. If, as above, they are recognising that it takes two to communicate, and they can take responsibility for the part they play, they may wish to write 'Learn to listen more', 'Improve communication skills' or 'Learn to be more independent'.

Achievements

List achievements the client is proud of positively, not 'I always fail at any new training I try to do'. Try 'At least I stuck that out for a year'. Other positive statements include: 'I found the strength to leave a bad job and look for a good one', 'I am always willing to tackle problems and take risks'. The achievements list is a great prompt to move you forward, because it focuses clients on the right questions, and keeps them positive and solution-oriented.

➤ What have I learnt from this?
➤ How have I progressed?
➤ What have I gained?
➤ How would I do things differently next time?

EXERCISE 6

Another way of working on goals is to identify your current position.

Write down the numbers 1 to 10 in a straight line. 1 is very negative, 10 is very positive. Circle the number that describes how you currently feel about your situation. This gives a statement of where you are to start working.

EXERCISE 7

List your personal core values. When we live in conflict with our inner values, it can lead to unhappiness, frustration and blocks. Becoming aware of your values and prioritising them helps you to reassess your goals.

➤ Start by making a list of 10 values that are important to you. Some common examples include: love, security, respect, money, achievement, health, success, ambition, freedom, integrity, compassion, independence, family, children, travel, trust.

➤ Next, try to put your own values in order, from 1 to 10. This can be difficult, and you may need to rework your list a few times before you feel it really reflects how you think and feel. Once you have done that, look at what the list is telling you. For example, if security, commitment and loyalty are high on your list, and you are working on short-term contracts, you are behaving in opposition to your values, and it will never make you happy. If freedom, independence and achievement are high on your list, you will need to be in a job that can give these qualities.

➤ Compare this list with your life now, or how you are planning your life. Are you living your life as you should? Are you planning your life with integrity?

Finding solutions

There are many ways to find solutions; and the solution is often there already, just hidden from view. Here are some options.

1 One way is to keep the focus on your own place in the problem. As above, focus on your own reaction, instead of blaming others. Then you are controlling both the problem and the solution. Ask yourself positive, self-focused and solution-focused questions: 'How can I ask questions in a way that X doesn't find threatening?'

2 If you find it difficult to see a way past the problem, try the doorway technique where you 'storm' every solution. Close your eyes and imagine each solution written on a doorway. Stand in front of one of the doors and walk through it. What is on the other side? If you do not like it, you can walk back through the door and try another one. Visualisation can be an unnerving but very powerful tool which helps you to see just what you most fear from making a particular decision. Using visualisation lets you walk through the doors again and again, until it looks less threatening. Keep asking yourself the right questions. 'How can I make this work for me?', 'How can I turn this situation around?'

3 Storm some solutions to long-standing problems.

⬇

Then write down any that, in retrospect, you feel would work.

⬇

Write down those that you would not consider.

⬇

Are there any left over that you are not sure about? Do not dismiss them. Make a note of them here and come back to them at a later date.

4 | **Write or draw the consequences** of some of the solutions you are considering. If drawing, use symbols such as animals or a situation – a ski run, a boat race – and place yourself and others at the heart of the solution.

5 Think of any random solution to a problem. The items can be as large or small as you wish – use them to form a checklist of things done/things to do.

Final steps

To complete the task, try the following exercise.

EXERCISE 8

List all the things you would like to achieve over your lifetime.
List those you could reasonably achieve within 10 years.
List those you will achieve this year.

Once you have identified your priorities, cost them and stage them, marking each target with an aim (what the plan is) and objective (how to map the outcome).

➤ Detail any targets for the year to come.

➤ Note how success will be measured once the object has been achieved.

➤ Note who is responsible for achieving it and by when, using basic *Who *Why *What *Where *When headings. Note the cost, if any, of your plan, and when you hope to achieve it by.

➤ Be specific and clear about the objectives.

Having defined your goals and planned their implementation, the next step is to audit your success in meeting them. Be proud of yourself and your achievements.

What are you currently doing towards meeting your present goal?
What do you plan to do next year?

SUMMARY

Having completed this chapter and worked through the exercises in the book, I hope you have a sense of improved self-awareness and self-knowledge. The book aimed to develop your individual strengths and talents, and help you to identify and improve your potential and personal autonomy. Assertiveness helps us fulfil aspirations. Personal development is also about establishing identity; developing competence, purpose and integrity and mature interpersonal relationships; managing emotions; and achieving interdependence.

You will now understand what assertiveness is and the skills needed to become assertive. You will have explored some of the clinical challenges: broadening your understanding of patient rights and the relevance of this in the new healthcare climate of patient empowerment. You will have learned how to manage conflict and aggression and how to break difficult news with understanding, expertise and compassion. We discussed setting boundaries in treatment, informing patients of their choices and also what we can and cannot be expected to deliver. We examined some of the models for working with this (care pathways, care planning, care aims, etc.) and how to develop our own communication skills and support patients with their learning. In this last section we explored how to use assertion skills in setting goals for ourselves and our clients and managing the process of change.

You will have learnt how you can apply assertiveness skills to develop yourself and your relationships with your colleagues and patients at work. You will have learnt how to manage yourself more effectively and, hopefully, how to be a more informed and effective worker within the ever-changing world of health, and social, care.

If you know yourself and understand others better, you are more likely to be able to take control of your life, and live it actively rather than passively. As you take on more responsibility, a different kind of respect is demanded which has intellectual, spiritual, personal, psychological and emotional implications. You will be ready to move on and up.

KEY POINTS

➤ Those who succeed will be those who have actively prepared for change.

➤ 'Good' change occurs when there is a clear sense of direction.

➤ To develop, people need to be experimental, creative, flexible and prepared to take risks.

➤ Change is a constant in the world. To survive – and grow – we must adjust to change. We need to understand that resistance to change is often the expression of insecurity and fear, as security is bedded in the past.

➤ Change has to be managed, and as with any management process it needs to be understood before it can be managed. We need to understand how to plan for, implement and evaluate it. We need to understand the forces driving change and our own reactions to it, and measure the size and shape of the work to be done.

➤ Change is always problematic because it presents dilemmas and conflict, so balances need to be struck, without compromising principles.

➤ Goals help develop individual commitment and reduce uncertainty in decision making, and help us to focus direction.
➤ Goal analysis means unpicking strengths, identifying immediate challenges/blocks/problems and development skills and achievements.
➤ Becoming aware of your core values and prioritising them helps you to assess your goals.

➤ List all the things you would like to achieve over your lifetime.
➤ List those you could reasonably achieve within 10 years.
➤ List those you will achieve this year.
➤ Audit your success.
➤ What are you currently doing towards meeting your present goal? What do you plan to do next year?

FURTHER READING

Halacre A. *First, Know What You Want – why goals don't work and how to make them.* Book Shaker; 2011.

Hayes J. *The Theory and Practice of Change Management.* 3rd ed. Palgrave Macmillan; 2010.

Latham GP. *Work Motivation: history, theory, research, and practice.* 2nd ed. Sage; 2012.

Mayne B. *Mapping: how to turn your dreams into realities.* Watkins Publishing; 2006.

Newton R. *Managing Change Step by Step: all you need to build a plan and make it happen.* Pearson Education; 2007.

Index

CPD with Radcliffe

You can now use a selection of our books to achieve CPD (Continuing Professional Development) points through directed reading.

We provide a free online form and downloadable certificate for your appraisal portfolio. Look for the CPD logo and register with us at: **www.radcliffehealth.com/cpd**

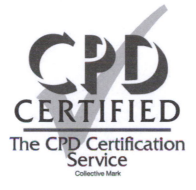